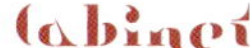

Cabinet

181 Wyckoff Street
Brooklyn NY 11217 USA
tel + 1 718 222 8434
fax + 1 718 222 3700
email info@cabinetmagazine.org
www.cabinetmagazine.org

Winter 2010–2011, issue 40

Editor-in-chief Sina Najafi
Senior editor Jeffrey Kastner
Editors D. Graham Burnett, Christopher Turner
UK editor Brian Dillon
Associate editor Claire Lehmann
Assistant editors Joshua Bauchner, Anya Kaplan-Seem
Art director Jessica Green
Website directors Ryan O'Toole, Luke Murphy
Editors-at-large Saul Anton, Mats Bigert, Brian Conley, Christoph Cox, Jesse Lerner, Jennifer Liese, Ryo Manabe, Alexander Nagel, Frances Richard, Daniel Rosenberg, Aaron Schuster, David Serlin, Debra Singer, Justin E. H. Smith, Margaret Sundell, Allen S. Weiss, Eyal Weizman, Margaret Wertheim, Gregory Williams, Jay Worthington, Tirdad Zolghadr
Contributing editors Molly Bleiden, Eric Bunge, Andrea Codrington, Pip Day, Charles Green, Carl Michael von Hausswolff, Adam Jasper, Srdjan Jovanovic Weiss, Dejan Krsic, Lytle Shaw, Cecilia Sjöholm, Sven-Olov Wallenstein
Editorial assistants Brian Miller, Anna Platt
Cabinet National Librarian Matthew Passmore

Printed in Belgium by the well-coiffed men and women of Die Keure.

Cabinet (USPS # 020-348, ISSN 1531-1430) is a quarterly magazine published by Immaterial Incorporated, 181 Wyckoff Street, Brooklyn, NY 11217. Periodicals Postage paid at Brooklyn, NY and additional mailing offices.

Postmaster
Please send address changes to Cabinet, 181 Wyckoff Street, Brooklyn, NY 11217.

Individual Subscriptions
1 year (4 issues): US $32, Canada $38, Western Europe $40, Elsewhere $50
2 years (8 issues): US $60, Canada $72, Western Europe $76, Elsewhere $96

Email subscriptions@cabinetmagazine.org or call + 1 718 222 8434.
Subscriptions address: 181 Wyckoff Street, Brooklyn, NY 11217, USA
Please either send a check in US dollars made out to "Cabinet," or mail, fax, or email us your Visa/MC/AmEx/Discover information. Subscriptions are also available online at www.cabinetmagazine.org/subscribe or through Paypal (paypal@cabinetmagazine.org).

Institutional Subscriptions
Institutional subscriptions available through EBSCO, Swets, or via our website.

Advertising
Email advertising@cabinetmagazine.org or call + 1 718 222 8434.

Distribution
Cabinet is available in the US and Canada through Disticor, which distributes both using its own network and through Ingram, Source Interlink, Armadillo News, Ubiquity, Hudson News, Small Changes, Last Gasp, Emma Marian Ltd, Cowley Distribution, Kent News, LMPI, MSolutions, The News Group, Don Olson Distribution, and Chris Stadler Distribution. If you'd like to use one of these distributors, contact Melanie Raucci at Disticor. Tel: + 1 631 587 1160, Email: mraucci@disticor.com.

Cabinet is available in Europe and elsewhere through Central Books, London. Email: orders@centralbooks.com.

Cabinet is available as a book (with an ISBN) through Distributed Arts Publishers (DAP). Tel: + 1 212 627 1999, Email: dap@dapinc.com.

Email us at circulation@cabinetmagazine.org or call + 1 718 222 8434 if you need further information.

Submissions
We only accept electronic submissions. See <www.cabinetmagazine.org/information/submissions.php> for guidelines. Please do not send any paper submissions.

Cabinet is a non-profit 501(c)(3) magazine published by Immaterial Incorporated. Our survival is dependent on support from generous foundations and individuals. Please consider supporting us at whatever level you can. Contributions are tax-deductible for those who deal with Uncle Sam. All gifts are acknowledged online; donations of $25 or more will be noted in the next possible issue, and those above $100 will be noted for four consecutive issues. Checks to "Cabinet" can be sent to our office; please write "This'll give you goosebumps" on the envelope.

Cabinet wishes to thank the following visionary foundations and individuals for their support of our activities during 2011. Additionally, we will forever be indebted to the extraordinary contribution of the Flora Family Foundation from 1999 to 2004; without their support, this publication would not exist. We would also like to extend our enormous gratitude to the Orphiflamme Foundation for their continued generous support.

$70,000
The Lambent Foundation

$50,000
The Andy Warhol Foundation for the Visual Arts

$20,000 – $25,000
The New York State Council on the Arts, The National Endowment for the Arts, Hesu Coue-Wilson & Edward Wilson

$10,000 – $14,999
The New York City Department of Cultural Affairs, The Greenwall Foundation

$5,000 – $9,999
Spencer Finch, Terry Winters

$2,500 – 3,500
Art Matters, The Danielson Foundation, Stina & Herant Katchadourian, Conor O'Neil

$1,000 – $2,000
Martha & Thomas G. Armstrong, Helen Bing, Christina & D. Graham Burnett, Paul Singh, Nina Zolt & Miles Gilburne

$500 or under
Tauba Auerbach, Tina Bennett, Margaret Holen, Deb Levy, Deborah Lovely, Jenna Lyons & Vincent Mazeau, Sara Meltzer Gallery, Lisa Moran, Jessica Wiederhorn, Debra Singer & Jay Worthington

$250 or under
Katerina Alexandraki, Defne Ayas, Anthony Aziz & Sammy Cucher, Elmira Bayrasli, Rachel Bers, Mathilde Billaud, Molly Bleiden & Scott Pfaffman, Alexis Bloom, Steve Bodow, Christine Chi, Emilie Clark & Lytle Shaw, Kristen Dodge, Cédric Duroux & Guy Walther, The Eagle family, Rebecca Lawton Flatters, Paul Fleming, George Ganat, Beverly & Wayne Gilbert, Karin Greene & Jaime Davidovich, Larissa Harris, Alexandra Hays, Mimi Hoang & Eric Bunge, Craig Kalpakjian, Lynn & James Karegeannes, James Katzenberger, Philippa Kaye, Jeannine Kiely, Melissa Landauer, Scott LeBouef , Kara Leibowitz, Cristina Linclau, Hugh Lynch, Machine Project, Carrington Madden, Chloe Malle, Roland Meerdter, Jenny Monick, Michael Morris, Paul Morris, Alexander Nagel, Pedram Navab, Jason Olin, Joshua Ramo, Clint Roenisch, Alison Rossiter, John Sargent, Jesse Shapins, Arlene Shechet & Mark Epstein, John Sherburne, Melanie Shorin & Greg Feldman, Brian Selznick & David Serlin, Mark Sheinkman, John Sherburne, Scott Tiede, Eugenie Tsai & Thomas Finkelpearl

$100 or under
Brian Cohen, Janelle Classen, Erika deVries, Cooper Downs, Peter Hussell, Maria Levistky, Craig Lucas, Brian Morgan, John Mozley, Michael Oldham, Nasrine Seraji

Cover: Julia Jacquette, *Blond Hair (Long)*, 2009. Photo Jean Vong.

Page 4: French miller Louis Coulon in 1904, sheltering a kitten in his cozy eleven-foot beard.

Erratum: In "Rock, Paper, Scissors" in issue 39, Kreuzberg was erroneously identified as a neighborhood in former East, rather than West, Berlin.

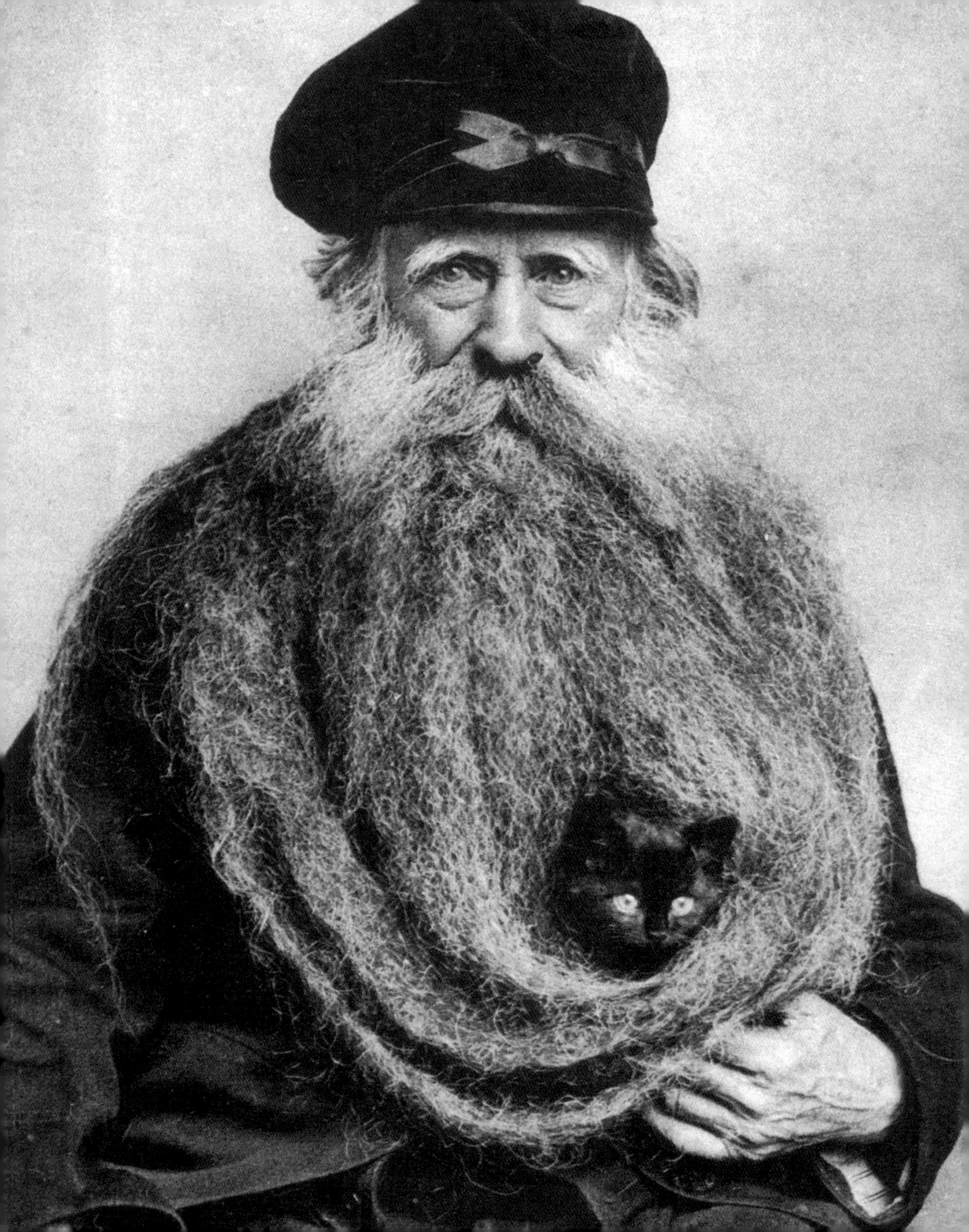

Janine Antoni is a Bahamian artist based in New York, who had her third solo exhibition at Luhring Augustine Gallery, New York, in 2009. Her work was included in "Move: Choreographing You" at the Hayward Gallery, London (2010), and will be seen in 2011 in "Heroines" at the Museo Thyssen-Bornemisza, Madrid, and "Dance/Draw" at the ICA, Boston.

Mats Bigert is an editor-at-large of *Cabinet*, and one half of the Swedish artist duo Bigert & Bergström.

Michael Bracewell is a writer based in London. Recent books include new editions of his novel *The Conclave* (Secker & Warburg, 1991/Capuchin Classics, 2010) and *England Is Mine* (Flamingo, 1997/Faber Finds, 2010).

Laurel Braitman is a historian and anthropologist of science currently completing her doctorate at MIT. Her book *Animal Madness* is forthcoming from Simon and Schuster.

D. Graham Burnett is an editor of *Cabinet* and teaches history of science at Princeton University.

Francis Cape is an artist working in Narrowsburg, New York. Projects in 2010 included *The Other End of the Line* at the High Line, New York, and "Behind the Levees," a summary of five years of post-Katrina work, at Colgate University's Clifford Gallery. Forthcoming in 2011 are exhibits based on Cape's 2009 series "Home Front" and a book of his New Orleans work.

Moyra Davey is a New York-based artist. In 2010, she had a solo exhibition at Kunsthalle Basel. Other recent group exhibitions include *Photography on Photography: Reflections on the Medium Since 1960* at the Metropolitan Museum of Art, New York (2008) and *Mixed Use Manhattan* at the Reina Sofia, Madrid (2010).

Brian Dillon is UK editor of *Cabinet* and an AHRC research fellow at the University of Kent. He is the author of *Tormented Hope: Nine Hypochondriac Lives* (Penguin, 2009) and a memoir, *In the Dark Room* (Penguin, 2005). His novel, *Sanctuary*, will be published by Sternberg Press in spring 2011.

Yara Flores is a designer and illustrator who writes on the history of visual culture and media. Originally from Brazil, she now lives in Puerto Rico.

Blake Gopnik is the chief art critic of the *Washington Post*. He is currently conducting research on eccentric perspective in Dutch art. His work can be seen at <www.blakegopnik.com>.

Sabrina Gschwandtner is a New York-based artist. Her work was recently included in "Hand+Made" at the Contemporary Arts Museum, Houston, and will be seen in the forthcoming exhibition "Shot Through" at Hordaland Art Centre, Norway.

Rachel Harrison is a New York–based artist. Her most recent monograph, *Museum With Walls*, was published on the occasion of the exhibitions "Consider the Lobster" at the Center for Curatorial Studies at Bard College, Annandale-on-Hudson, New York; "HAYCATION" at Portikus, Frankfurt; and "Conquest of the Useless" at Whitechapel Gallery, London.

Julia Jacquette is an artist based in New York. Her work is in the collections of the Museum of Modern Art, New York, and the Museum of Fine Arts, Boston, among others. Her next solo exhibition will take place in April 2011 at the Anna Kustera Gallery.

Wayne Koestenbaum is a Distinguished Professor at the CUNY Graduate Center in New York. He has published twelve books of poetry, criticism, and fiction, including, most recently, *Hotel Theory* (Soft Skull, 2007) and *Best-Selling Jewish Porn Films* (Turtle Point Press, 2006).

So Yoon Lym is a painter based in northern New Jersey. She had a solo exhibition, "The Dreamtime: Hair and Braid Pattern Paintings," in November 2010 at the Paterson Museum, New Jersey. Her next solo exhibition, "Urban Patterns," will take place in April 2011 at the Arthur M. Berger Gallery, Manhattanville College, Purchase, New York.

Emma Markiewicz works at the National Archives in London. She is currently completing a PhD dissertation titled "Hair, Wigs, and Wig Wearing in Eighteenth-Century England" at the University of Warwick.

Virgil Marti is a Philadelphia-based artist represented by the Elizabeth Dee Gallery, New York. "Set Pieces: Curated by Virgil Marti from the Collection of the Philadelphia Museum of Art" is on view through 13 February 2011 at the ICA, Philadelphia.

Meredith Martin is an assistant professor of art history at Wellesley College. Her book, *Dairy Queens: The Politics of Pastoral Architecture from Catherine de' Medici to Marie-Antoinette*, was just published by Harvard University Press (2011). Her new project concerns diplomatic relations between France and India in the eighteenth century.

Carol Mavor is professor in the Department of Art History and Visual Studies at the University of Manchester. She is the author of three books, including *Becoming: The Photographs of Clementina, Viscountess Hawarden* (1999) and *Pleasures Taken: Performances of Sexuality and Loss in Victorian Photographs* (1995), both published by Duke University Press. Currently, she is completing a series of short essays on the color blue to be published under the title *Blue Mythologies* (Reaktion Books, 2011).

Vik Muniz is an internationally exhibited artist based in Brooklyn and Rio de Janeiro. He is also involved in social projects that use artmaking as a force for change; his work with Brazilian garbage pickers was the focus of the award-winning 2010 documentary *Waste Land*. In collaboration with other artists, he is currently curating "The Art Week," an urban art intervention scheduled to take place in May 2011 throughout Rio de Janeiro.

Spyros Papapetros teaches art, architectural theory, and historiography in the School of Architecture and the Program in Media and Modernity at Princeton University. He is the editor of Siegfried Ebeling's *Space as Membrane* (AA Publications, 2010) and has completed a book-length study on turn-of-the-century discourses of animation (forthcoming in 2011).

Ester Partegàs is a Brooklyn-based artist. She holds an MFA in sculpture from Universitat de Barcelona and another in multimedia art from Universität der Künste, Berlin. Recent solo shows include "Less World" at Christopher Grimes Gallery, Santa Monica, and "More World" at Foxy Production, New York, both in 2010.

Aaron Schuster is a writer based in Berlin, where he is a fellow at the Institute for Cultural Inquiry. He completed a PhD in philosophy at the Katholieke Universiteit Leuven, Belgium, in 2010. He can be reached at <aaron_schuster@yahoo.com>.

Jorian Polis Schutz is a writer, publisher, and calligrapher living in Brooklyn, New York, and Boulder, Colorado. His publishing imprint, Orphiflamme Press, will release its first book, *Varitan's Illustrated Greek Myths*, in spring 2011.

William H. Sherman is director of the Centre for Renaissance & Early Modern Studies at the University of York, the author of *John Dee* (University of Massachusetts Press, 1995) and *Used Books* (University of Pennsylvania Press, 2007), and the editor of plays by Shakespeare, Jonson, and Marlowe. He is currently writing a book that he is trying not to call *The Bacon Code*.

Alexandre Singh is a Franco-British artist working in New York. His work is currently on view in "Free" at the New Museum, New York, and in "Manifesta 8" in Spain. He will be curating the spring 2011 issue of *Palais*, the magazine of the Palais de Tokyo, Paris.

Justin E. H. Smith teaches philosophy at Concordia University in Montreal. He is the author of *Divine Machines: Leibniz and the Sciences of Life* (Princeton University Press, 2011). His new book project is entitled *Nature, Human Nature, and Human Difference: Early Modern Natural Philosophy in Global Context, 1600–1800*.

Jane South is an artist based in Brooklyn, New York.

Christopher Turner is an editor of *Cabinet*. His book, *Adventures in the Orgasmatron: How the Sexual Revolution Came To America*, will be published by Farrar, Straus and Giroux in the US and by HarperCollins in the UK in June 2011.

Volker M. Welter teaches architectural history at the University of California at Santa Barbara. He is the author of *Biopolis: Patrick Geddes and the City of Life* (MIT Press, 2002). His book *Ernst L. Freud and the Case of the Modern Bourgeois Home*, a study of the work of the architect-son of Sigmund Freud, will be published by Berghahn Books in 2011.

COLORS / GOLD
MICHAEL BRACEWELL

Elvis stands with his feet spaced widely apart, his shoulders dropped, his arms hanging loosely. There is good-humored self-consciousness in the young King's demeanor, but what renders him regal, by way of the most immediate signifier on offer, is his suit (and bow-tie) of pure shining gold. By common assent, Elvis's reign is undisputed, and the gold suit—it looks as shiny as kitchen foil—is the garment that transforms him from commoner to monarch. The effect is more vaudevillian, almost clown-like, than rock-and-roll cool, but such is the iconic image on the cover of Presley's *50,000,000 Elvis Fans Can't Be Wrong*, released in 1959—just three years after his breakthrough single "Heartbreak Hotel" dominated the charts on both sides of the Atlantic— and in doing so arguably marked the beginning of the pop age as we know it.

Elvis's gold suit, for all its swagger, somehow lacks sex appeal. Glancing quickly, you might think that the King was wearing a rather extravagant pair of pajamas. It is a garment clearly descended from the ceremonial dinner suits worn by dance band musi-cians and theatrical entertainers—although Elvis's pride in being an "entertainer" would remain one of his most endearing qualities. (Later, when fat, imperial, and high on kung fu, Elvis would be asked at a press conference what he thought about US involvement in Vietnam. "Ah'm sorry suh," he mumbled back, "but ah'm jus' an entertainer.") Back in 1959, however, the totality of the suit's gold, its sheer slab-like shim-mer—more TV game show than Versailles—asserted a pop Americana update of Shakespeare's oft-quoted comment on style and kingship: "My presence, like a robe pontifical, ne'er seen but wonder'd at."

For *50,000,000 Elvis Fans Can't Be Wrong*, Pres-ley was suited in gold by the wonderfully named Nudie Cohn—whose own story, as the King's tailor, reads like a glamorously American reclamation of a European fairy tale. Nudie had arrived in New York in the 1940s, and started a business making "undergarments for showgirls"—an occupation which one somehow imag-ines being Groucho Marx's dream job. "Nudies for the Ladies" was a fair success, but it was only later, after a country singer called Tex Williams bought Nudie a sewing machine from the proceeds of an auctioned horse, that "Nudies Rodeo Tailors" was born in North Hollywood to provide rhinestones and fringes to the aristocracy of American music. (Some forty-five years after Cohn created Elvis's look for his 1959 album, Mark

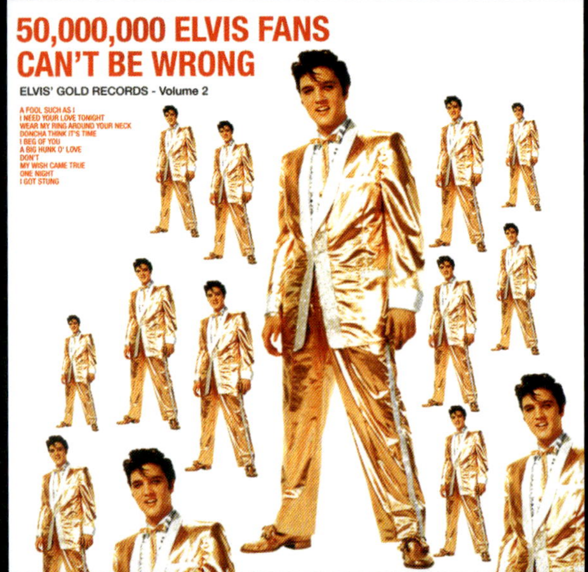

Elvis Presley, *50,000,000 Elvis Fans Can't Be Wrong*, 1959.

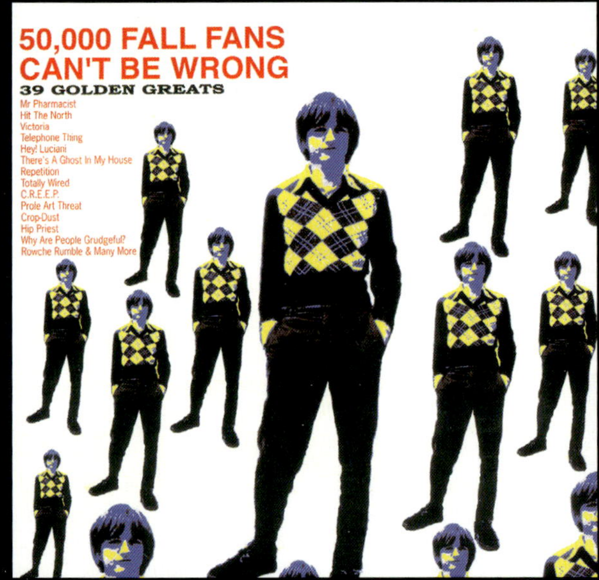

The Fall, *50,000 Fall Fans Can't Be Wrong*, 2004.

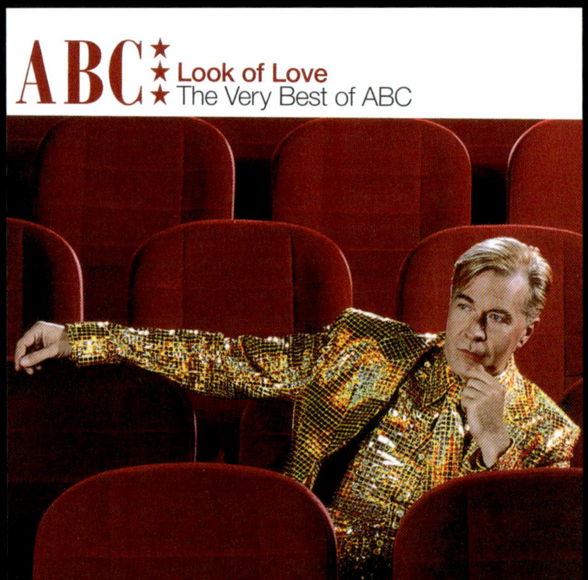

ABC, *Look of Love*, 2002.

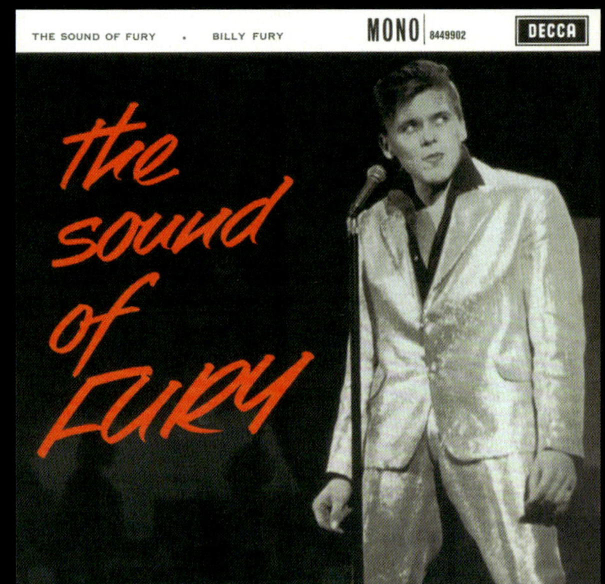

Billy Fury, *The Sound of Fury*, 1960.

E. Smith—ever pop's republican—would be found on the cover of *50,000 Fall Fans Can't Be Wrong* with the kingly gold suit replaced by sweater and jeans.)

In terms of myth, Nudie Cohn's gold suit for Elvis can be seen as the beginning of a lineage—the creation of a mantle to pass down, and the inauguration of gold as an archetypal aspect of pop iconography. Fast-forward a year and cross the Atlantic to Liverpool, where Billy Fury—"The Elvis of Birkenhead"—has just recorded his signature album, *The Sound of Fury*. Released in 1960 on the Decca label (they who would turn down the Beatles) and destined (unfairly) to reach only number eighteen on the UK Top Twenty, *The Sound of Fury* remains distinguished as a great British Beat album mostly by way of its cover artwork. Now it's Fury wearing a (or "the") gold suit—this time with a black shirt—and somehow he looks cooler and sharper than the King himself. It is as though the gold suit has lost the stiffness of its newness, becoming worn-in and slick. It has also become strangely Anglicized—less brash and loud—even though the entire universe it celebrates is primarily black American.

Combine the stage name Billy Fury with the ceremonial pop mantle of the gold suit and you have a virtually pure pop statement—up there with Johnny's leather jacket in *The Wild Ones* or Johnny Ray's hearing-aid or Lord Byron's club foot. Gold—oft reputed, like diamonds, to curse those who crave it—is both an alchemical substance (that which has been refined, leaving behind the dross) and capable of conducting a current, a useful capacity in a medium which, to quote Patti Smith, is the (un)natural consequence of "Art + Electricity." But might pop's gold suit be haunted—fable-like, bestowing fame, wealth, and glamour in exchange for long life, and even soul? (British artist Linder's recent performance work and film, *The Dark Town Cake Walk: Celebrated from the House of FAME* (2010), enacts this exchange, delivering on cue the archetype of the Star—clad in gold lamé—who is placed in sacrificial configuration with the archetype of the Witch; Linder's point being the relationship between glamour and magic.)

And so: Elvis dead of heart failure by 1977; likewise, tragically, Billy Fury by 1983—the year New Romanticism morphed into the soundtrack of Yuppie dreams of *la vie deluxe* by way of Spandau Ballet's UK number two hit, "Gold," with its exhortation to "always believe in your soul." (Meanwhile, if you go to Liverpool's great Anglican cathedral, pop fans, you'll discover in the choir there a simple oak lectern with the name "BILLY FURY" inscribed in gold—a conflation of faiths that is hard to resist, remake, or remodel.) With his usual acuity, British style analyst Peter York would subsequently note the manner in which the trajectory of New Romanticism would keep in perfect step with the rise of Thatcherite ideology—"Gold," in all its triumphalism, was the perfect song for the new generation of venture capitalists with smooth jaws, clean arteries, and fat pens.

But the gold suit—untamed—dances down the decades. In 1973, for example, we find the young Malcolm McDowell starring in *O Lucky Man!*, Lindsay Anderson's relentlessly cynical update of *A Pilgrim's Progress*. The suit is fitted for him by a fellow resident in a seedy hotel, who appears to be as much an agent of destiny or emissary of fate as the Hotel Manager in Benjamin Britten's operatic version of *Death in Venice*. McDowell wears the suit as though it were Arthurian armor—or as though it shared, with profound irony, a mid-Victorian, Anglo-Christian interpretation of Arthurian virtues. But still it cannot protect him. We see him plunging through Arcadian English countryside, soon to blunder into a horrific "research facility."

The magical aspect of glamour is unsurprisingly volatile, and pop's gold suit, even as it appears to empower and enshrine, also seems to bring with it the sin of hubris ("insolent pride towards the gods,") that seldom goes unpunished by the vagaries of mortality. Marc Bolan, Malcolm McLaren, and Morrissey will all triumph on pop's stage in shining gold—yet each has (or had) more than a nodding acquaintance with the shadow. In this, we might look upon pop's golden raiment as articulating, with a precision that is almost too neat, the dynamics of classic myth: ambition, triumph, irony, and tragedy. So always believe in your soul.

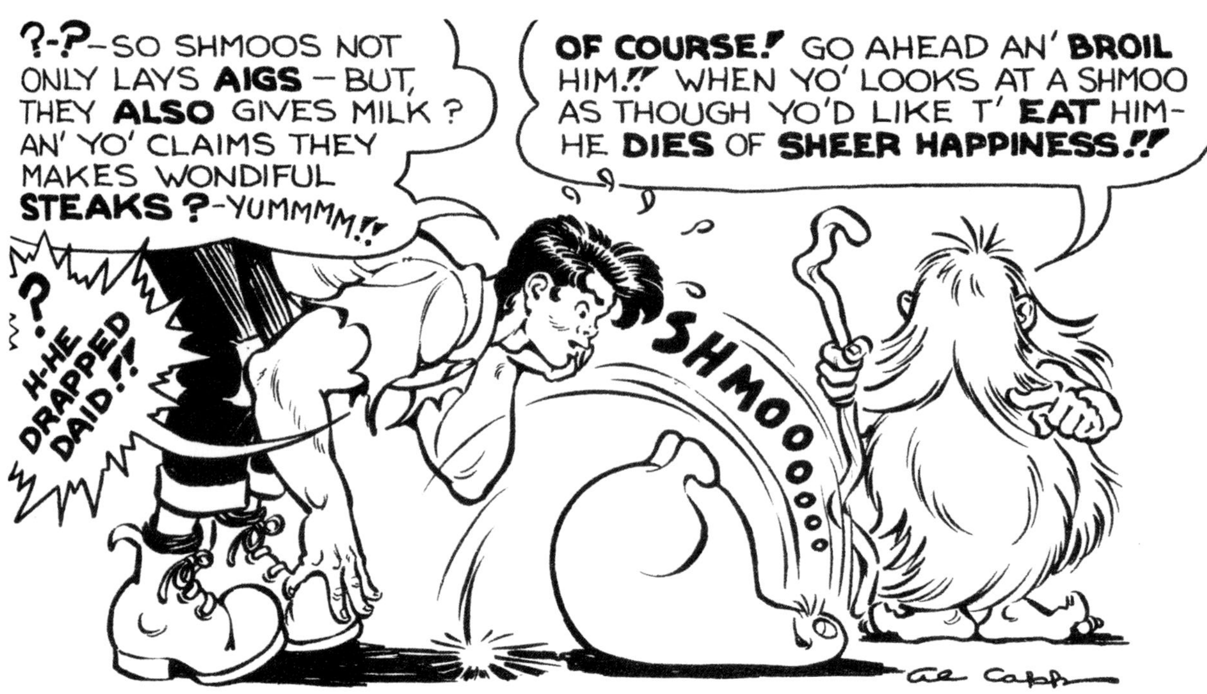

INGESTION / DIALECTICS OF THE SHMOO
YARA FLORES

I take as my text Al Capp's 1948 *The Life and Times of the Shmoo*, the book-form reprinting of Capp's original sequence of *L'il Abner* cartoons that, starting in August of that year, introduced American newspaper readers to the friendly, soft, colorless, gourd-shaped creature called the Shmoo.

A little context: the caustic, well-read, one-legged Capp (born Alfred Caplin, to a family of Russian Jewish descent then resident in New Haven, Connecticut) was, by 1948, a national figure on account of more than a decade of sardonic, exuberant, and irreverent cartooning. His nationally syndicated *L'il Abner* strip—depicting the hillbilly antics of the dirt-poor residents of Dogpatch, USA—had upwards of thirty million daily readers in the immediate postwar years, a number that would double in the decade to come. A febrile eroticist (whose work exudes an odor of adolescent incontinence), a savage social critic (whose indiscriminant satires convey something of the thin misanthropy of the crank), and a celebrity controversialist (whose clowning, camera-loving truculence foreshadowed features of our current media climate), Capp is an acquired taste. And it tastes a great deal like the 1950s. Steinbeck thought he was the greatest writer in America; that right there may

say it all. An admiring Updike called it all "Voltairean." One encounters allusions to Rabelais. Perhaps.

My Capp misgivings aside, it cannot be denied that the Shmoo represents a satirical conjuration of Swiftian proportions. Waylaid in the woods, the strip's eponymous hero (L'il Abner himself, a hunkish lout of good heart and little mind), stumbles upon the Valley of the Shmoo (guarded by a buxom Amazon, but never mind), where he discovers these impossibly friendly critters, whose unique desire, it would seem, is to give themselves up for human happiness. They lay eggs, give milk, and their flesh is sweet, approximating chicken when fried and steak when broiled. They are wholly boneless, reproduce every few minutes (apparently asexually, but I will return to this), and require zero upkeep. Most peculiarly expressive of their appetite for service, as L'il Abner soon discovers, is their propensity to die, spontaneously, when looked at with hunger. Overcome by affection for its new friend, one Shmoo lays a *cheesecake*.

The unfolding plotline brings out the critical edge of this fantasy creature from the land of Cockaigne: L'il Abner introduces the Shmoos to Dogpatch, where they instantly wreck the system of exploitative capitalism under which the Dogpatchers live. The bloodsucking grocer is bankrupted (yes, ugly anti-Semitic gestures are

---

All images from Al Capp, *The Life and Times of the Shmoo*, 1948.

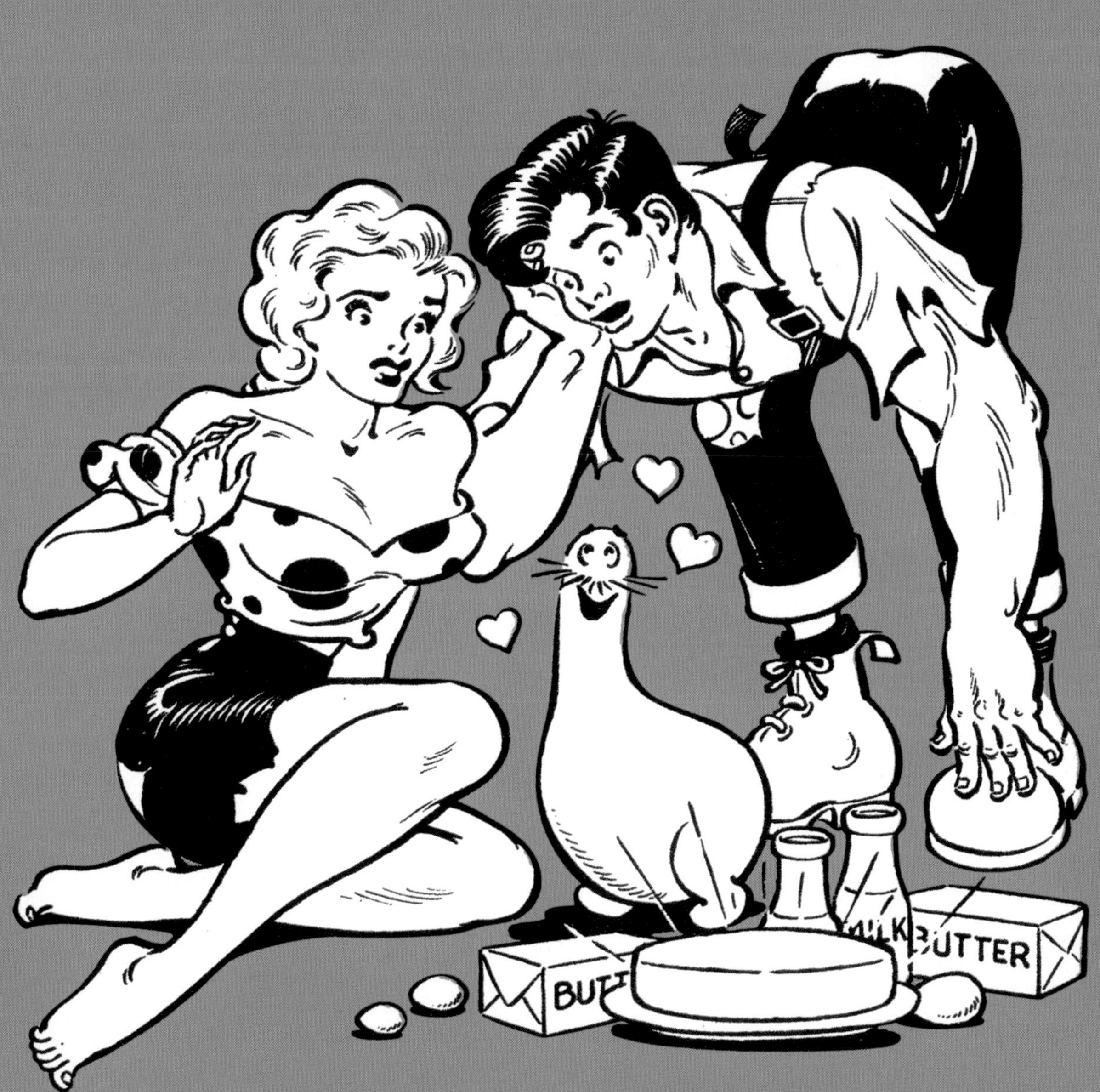
BUTTER
MILK
BUTTER

made here). The pork baron sees ruin on the horizon.
The factory industrialists cannot find wage labor. As this
"plague" of plenty spreads across the country, the forces
of reaction seize upon the magnitude of the crisis, hiring
an army of toughs to exterminate the Shmoos. In which
they are nearly successful: the Dogpatchers preserve
two, male and female, and sequel dramas hinge on the
question of restoring the race (note the contradiction
with Capp's presentation of the Shmoo as reproducing
via spontaneous "budding"—this is never worked out).

That a "Shmoo Craze" swept the nation between
1948 and 1952 is elsewhere documented. The creatures
and their creator made the cover of *Time* magazine.
Facsimile Shmoos were mobilized in the Berlin Airlift.
Shmoo licensing and products raised staggering sums
of money, upwards of twenty-five million (1948) dollars.

What concerns me here, however, is a brief resumé
of the critical uses of the Shmoo. Predictably, the left
has seen in *The Life and Times of the Shmoo* a visionary
parable of the contradictions of capitalism. In his valu-
able *Class Counts*, the distinguished Marxist sociologist
Erik Olin Wright (building on a suggestion by the British
philosopher G. A. Cohen) elaborates the core principles
of historical materialism using the Shmoo, reading *L'il
Abner* to explicate class interest and formally define
exploitation. Surprisingly, perhaps, others have inter-
preted the story the other way around, with Gary Wills,
for instance, seeing in the Shmoos a send-up of progressive social policies—a reading, in my view, difficult to
square with Capp's own Shmoo glosses from the late
1940s, which are pastoral in the extreme, and possess
something of the agrarian romanticism of early E. P.
Thompson (e.g., Capp on the inspiration for the Shmoo:
"the earth ... it's eager to give us everything we need"). It
is notoriously the case, however, that Capp did meander
to the right across the 1960s, emerging as a strident
hippy-basher and paleo-conservative. He may well have
repurposed the Shmoo across his own political evolution.

Although Capp himself made at best a middlebrow
feminist (and probably not even that), there have been
a few sympathetic gender-readings of the Shmoo (key
evidence: one of the original cartoons depicts a showgirl
no longer required to entertain her beau for a decent
meal). Wright himself notes in passing that housewives
are, from a patriarchal microeconomic perspective,
the original "Shmoo"—a something for nothing. On the
other hand, considerably more arresting is Greta Gaard's
suggestion that, in light of Carol J. Adams's *The Sexual
Politics of Meat*, the Shmoo must be understood as nothing less than carnivore porn: just as pornography norms
rape as the apotheosis of female desire, the Shmoo's

self-immolation whitewashes the grotesque violence of
the abattoir with a fantasy of meat-*jouissance*.

Shades of Bataille. And it is here, I think, that
we come to crux of the matter. Political-economic
readings of the Shmoos overlook—perhaps because
they must—the exquisite act of incandescent, spontaneous, erotic *autolysis* that lies at the real center of
the Shmoos' transgressive power: they are literally
consumed by love. They die of desire to feed their
flock. This is *self-sacrifice as transcendence*—the
absolute unspeakable of rational analysis, if also
the perennial matrix of human community.

The Shmoo: *materia prima* of the social body; the
Eucharist of utopia.

On 8 April 1747, Monsieur Garion, a blind wigmaker, sat on a stool in nervous anticipation. A man standing behind him held his head steady, one hand firmly under Garion's chin, the other peeling back the upper lid of his eye. Surgeon Jacques Daviel sat in front of them on a slightly higher chair and held down Garion's lower lid. Steadying his elbow on his knee, Daviel brought a sharp triangular-shaped knife up to the wigmaker's clouded eye and, without anaesthetic, pierced the cornea. Using another curved cutting knife and convex scissors, this wound was opened to create and lift a half-moon-shaped flap. A sharp needle was applied directly to the lens; any adhesions between it and the iris were severed with a blunt spatula. As fluid flowed out of the eye, gentle pressure was applied to the lower lid to help dislodge and remove the patient's cataract.

This was the first extracapsular cataract extraction operation on record. It was a seemingly miraculous procedure: when his bandages were removed after a week of bed rest, Garion could see again. Over the next forty years, Daviel performed 206 such operations, 182 of which he claimed were successful—impressive odds for the time. After he explained his method to the Académie Royale de Chirurgie in 1753, other surgeons followed suit. Over the next century, hundreds of different medical knives were designed to try to create smoother incisions, which would speed healing and minimalize the chance of infection. Surgeons developed their own signature cuts, and ophthalmology illustrations show a variety of these marks, scarred onto the cornea like runic signs or the Utopian alphabet invented by Thomas More. In one example, the doctors' surnames and the date of each procedure are inscribed below a circle containing their patented triangle, zigzag, anchor, square, cross, circle, or V and T slit. Together they form a secret language of eyes.

Eighteenth-century philosophers were fascinated by blindness—Locke, Leibniz, La Mettrie, Diderot, and Voltaire were all interested in the intellectual problems thrown up by the new science, or art, of cataract surgery. The blind man restored to sight became a paradigmatic figure in Enlightenment thinking. "To rediscover the permanent truth of this bright, distant, open naivety of the gaze" was, according to Michel Foucault, one of the "great mythical experiences on which the philosophy of the eighteenth century had wished to base its beginning."

In 1688 the Irish scientist and politician William Molyneux, whose wife lost her sight in the first

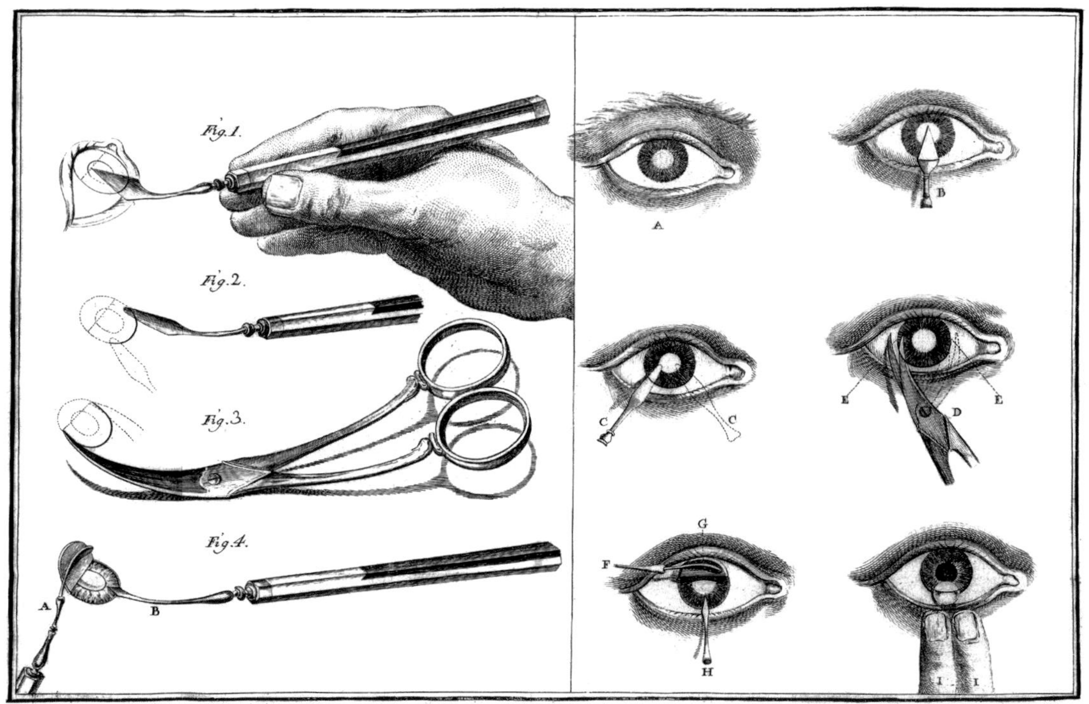

Instruments used in cataract operations. From a 1780 edition of Johannes de Gorter's *Cirugia expurgada*. Courtesy Wellcome Library.

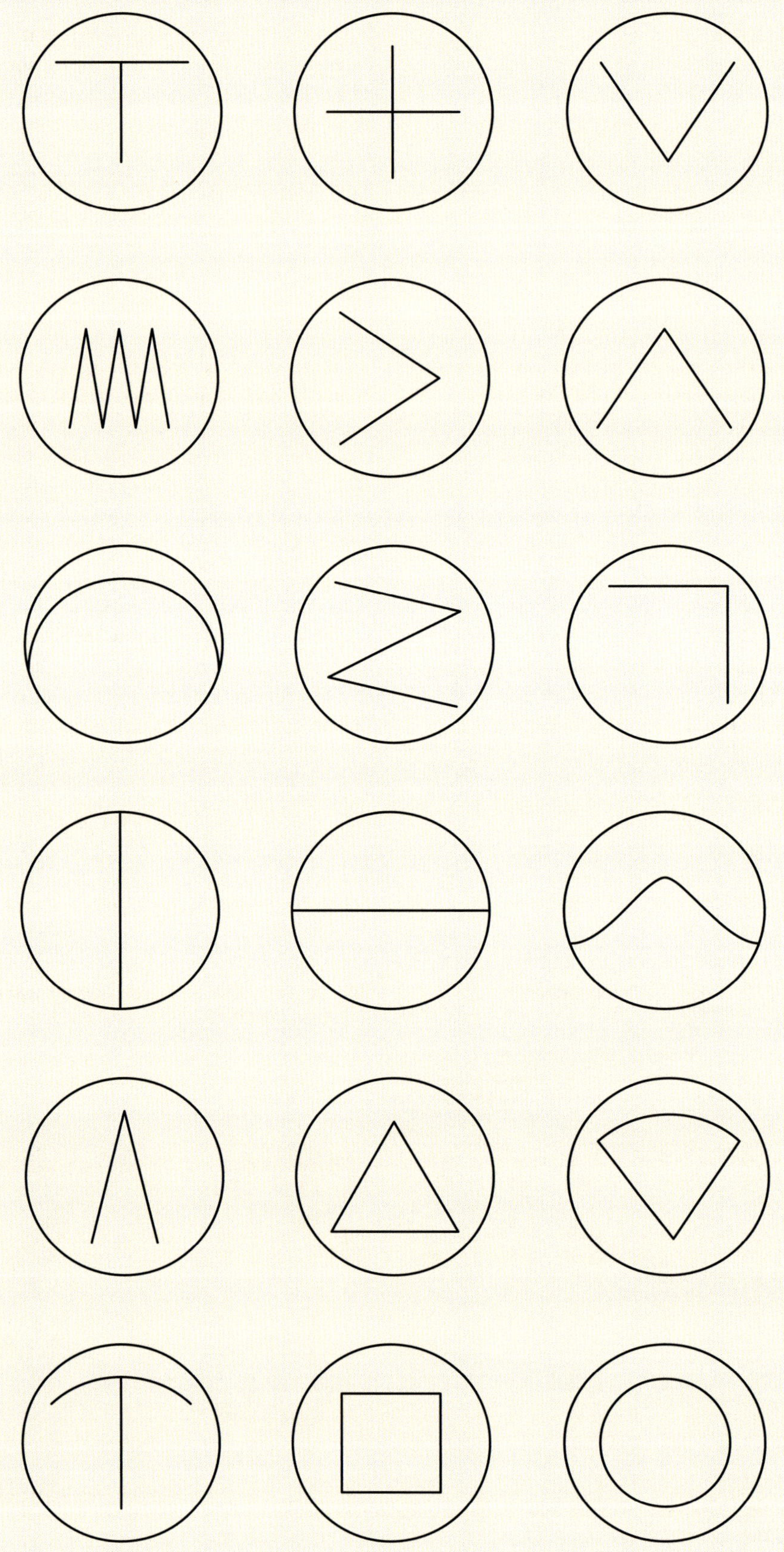

year of their marriage, posed a question to John Locke: would a man born blind, who has learned to distinguish objects by touch, be able to distinguish a globe and a cube by sight alone if he were ever cured? After Locke wrote about it in 1690 in his *Essay Concerning Human Understanding*, philosophers grappled with what came to be known as the Molyneux problem. However, it was only in 1728, when the London surgeon William Cheselden operated on a thirteen-year-old boy, removing the cataracts that had made him blind soon after birth, that Molyneux's thought experiment could be practically tested.

Cheselden, working before Daviel's pioneering surgery, used a method known as "couching" to push the opaque lens from the line of vision with a special needle. This method had been practiced, with minimal success, since antiquity. The lens, rather than the retina, was thought to be the vehicle of sight and the cataract (from *cataracta*, Latin for waterfall) a coagulated obstruction between it and the pupil. Though physicians misunderstood the role of the lens in vision, by working the hardened, or "ripe," cataract away from the pupil with a sharp point, pushing it to the back of the eye or breaking it into pieces, vision could be restored.

The Cheselden boy's "conversion" to sight (attended by a local minister) was described in almost biblical terms: "When the patient first received the dawn of light there appeared such ecstasy in his action that he seemed ready to swoon away in the surprise of joy and wonder," wrote one witness to the patient's Damascus moment. In the sensory confusion of first sight, the boy had no spatial sense and "thought all objects whatever touch'd his eyes." Molyneux's problem was therefore answered in the negative—the boy couldn't distinguish a cube and sphere without testing them first with his hands (he had to learn to see)—but the debate still raged. Was the boy asked leading questions? Had he been given time to recover from the operation? Was he intelligent enough?

Surgeons were keen to replicate Cheselden's success and contribute to this philosophical discussion. However, eye surgery, with its promise of dramatic cures, remained a controversial field. Operations were often performed by itinerant barber surgeons, rogue oculists who would travel across Europe and as far as Russia and Persia, performing these dangerous procedures before large audiences in the central squares of towns. One such quack doctor, John Taylor, who had in fact been trained by Cheselden at St. Thomas's Hospital in London, would arrive in a carriage painted with pictures of eyeballs and the motto: *"Qui dat videre dat viver"* (He who gives sight, gives life).

Taylor treated people from all social strata, and claimed to have cured emperors, popes, and kings (including George II). It was lucrative work: if people couldn't pay his exorbitant fees, he accepted valuables, such as gold fob watches, instead. He distributed handbills that lauded him as "Chevalier" and "Ophthalmiater Royal" and used flamboyant, occult techniques, such as administering eye drops created from the blood of slaughtered pigeons. The French surgeon Pierre Guérin described how Taylor would bind his patients' couched eyes with gauze that included egg white, baked apple, or salt, and sometimes a coin: "He would exalt; he would proclaim a miracle; he plugged the eye with firm recommendation not to uncover it until after five or six days, and he left on the fourth, after having exploited the victims of his bad faith."

In 1750, Taylor operated on the sixty-six-year-old Johann Sebastian Bach in Leipzig. On this occasion, Taylor was still around when the composer's bandages were removed a week later. Having failed to restore his sight, Taylor operated on Bach's eyes a second time and administered mercury treatment and bleeding. Rendered completely blind, and in terrible pain, Bach died a few months after his surgery from a post-operative infection. Eight years later, Taylor operated on George Frideric Handel in London with similar lack of success. Handel, who had already undergone several couching operations, spent the last decade of his life in darkness. He would cry as he listened to the aria from his oratorio, *Samson* (1741): "Total eclipse: no sun, no moon, all dark amidst the blaze of noon."

Jacques Daviel's newly invented technique, which might have saved Handel's vision, gave some much needed legitimacy to eye surgery and remained the predominant technique until the 1950s, when ophthalmologists began inserting artificial lenses into the eye; now technological developments and prosthetics such as laser surgery, retinal simulators, and touch-sight devices offer new hope to the long-term blind. While a few charlatan cataract cutters replaced them, couching quacks like Taylor went out of business in the late eighteenth century. Taylor died in obscurity; with poetic justice, and like his many victims, he also died blind. Samuel Johnson liked to cite his career as a cautionary tale, an example of "how far impudence may carry ignorance."

---

opposite: A sample of signature lens incisions used by different surgeons in the nineteenth century. From Marvin L. Kwitko and Charles D. Kelman, *The History of Modern Cataract Surgery*, 1998.

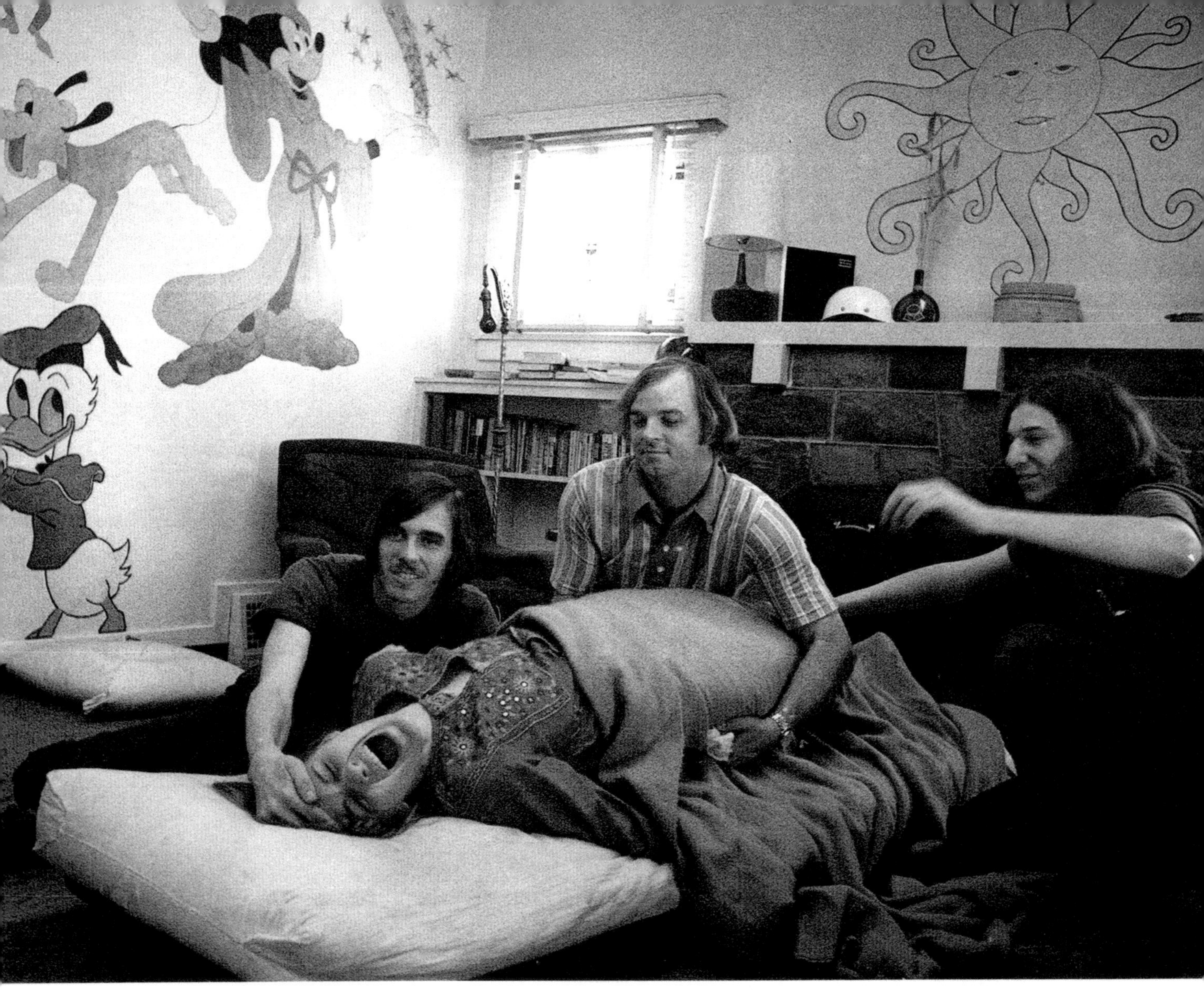

LEGEND / RESTRAINT
WAYNE KOESTENBAUM

Art requires restraint. Too much emotion, too many liberties taken, and the work falls apart.

The artist alone can't supply the restraint. Outside forms must save the artist from the peril of excessive emotion.

The artist, if lucky, has friends—severe friends, who can corral the artist's wayward instincts and provide closure, symmetry, irony.

Without restraint, an artist might fall into the bathetic, the regressive; without restraint, the artist might return to the sad level of a Donald Duck, a Mickey Mouse, a Pluto.

Baudelaire nearly outgrew the alexandrine; he fought against it. But the alexandrine won. The alexandrine tied Baudelaire to his bed. Baudelaire screamed. Baudelaire's spine arched. Baudelaire remembered visiting the Salpêtrière; he remembered the florid antics of the ill and the mad. Baudelaire begged the alexandrine, "Have mercy!" Baudelaire, like a lesbian, or a sphinx, or a legendary beauty in her palace, smiled, his mouth open, teeth flashing, tongue glistening, like the voluptuous furniture, polished by the years, surrounding him.

Mickey Dolenz, lead vocalist in the Monkees, also knew restraint, and reaped rewards from it. Without the restraint of a song's form, how could "Randy Scouse Git" have been born? The same goes for "Going Down," or "Regional Girl." Without the restraints—temporal, syntactic, stylistic—of a pop song's armature, how could "Shorty Blackwell" have hit the big time?

Mickey Dolenz's cuteness, too, blossomed under the harsh sign of Restraint. If Mickey Dolenz had relaxed into the randomly effeminate or the chunkily pugilistic, his aesthetic appeal would never have risen like a burning comet in TV's azure. Because of situation comedy's restraints, and because of the limits that Masculinity, as a sign system, imposed on his behavior, Mickey was able to achieve a cuteness that we can only compare to Baudelaire's use of the sonnet form; though it is doubtful that a poem like "La Beauté" ("*Je suis belle, ô mortels! comme un rêve de pierre*") physically stimulates its readers, the effect of its closely spaced rhymes and rigidly limited lexicon on the limbic system has much in common with the arousing effect that Mickey's body, in its prime, produced in the teen spectator.

If restraints did not exist in art, we would not have Jeff Koons's photographs of himself in sexual intercourse with his then-wife Cicciolina, an Italian porn star. Only the conventions of photography, as a medium blessed with restraint, allowed these images to attain parturition. We could say, courting pomposity, that restraint allowed Jeff Koons's erect penis, whether simulated or real, to cross the proscenium of art, to leave behind the childish world of experience, and to enter representation, with its salutary illusions, codes, abrasions, and liqueurs.

Therefore, too, we are in the position of thanking restraint for its brute force. We thank restraint for its muscular arms, its wristwatch, its moustache; we thank restraint for its unventilated parlor, its lack of deodorant, its athlete's foot, its dandruff; we thank restraint for its unclipped fingernails, its dirty kleenexes, its dingleberries. To restraint, we bow down; we lick the soles of restraint's brogues.

MAIN

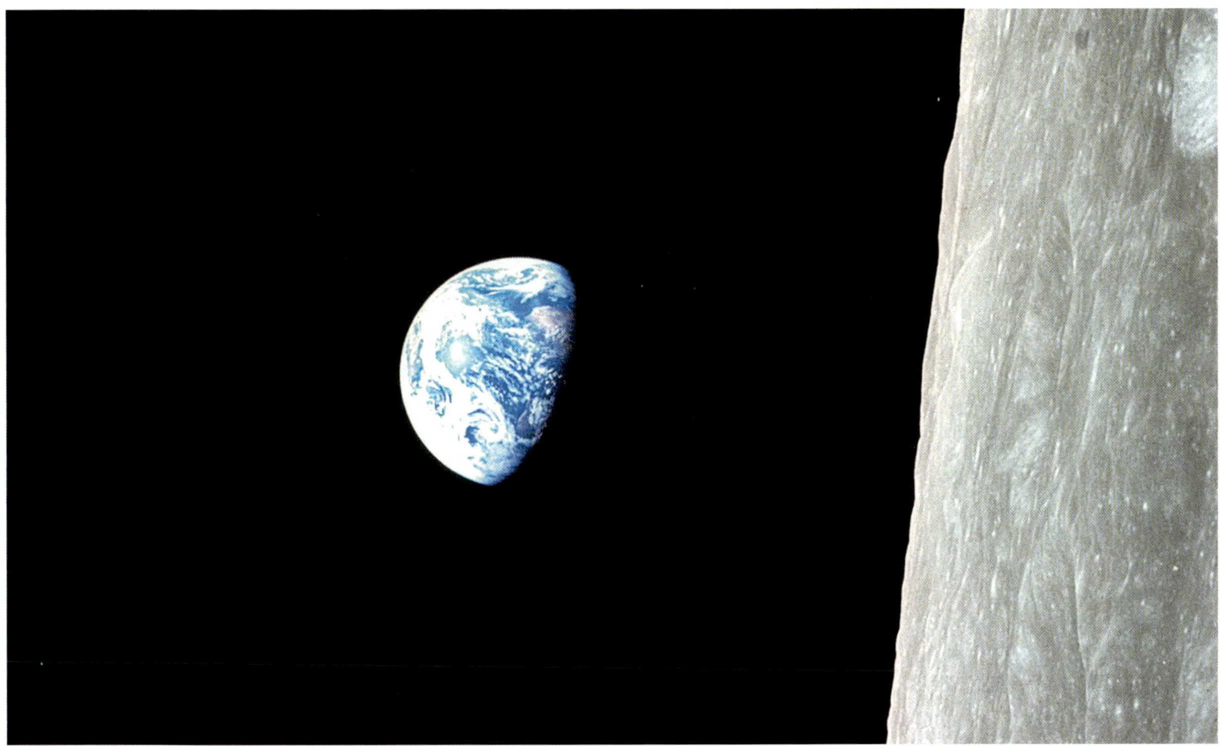

"Earthrise," photographed by *Apollo 8* on 12 December 1968. According to NASA, "this view of the rising Earth … is displayed here in its original orientation, though it is more commonly viewed with the lunar surface at the bottom of the photo."

FROM DISC TO SPHERE
VOLKER M. WELTER

In October 1969, at the height of the irrational fears about the imminent detonation of the population bomb, about one hundred hippies assembled in the San Francisco Bay area to stage a "hunger show," a week-long period of total fasting. The event was inspired by a hashish-induced vision that had come to the founder of the *Whole Earth Catalog*, Stewart Brand, when reading Paul Ehrlich's 1968 book *The Population Bomb*. The goal was to personally experience the bodily pain of those who suffer from famine and to issue a warning about the mass starvations predicted for the 1970s. From the outset, the lofty intentions conflicted with a more dreary reality. Originally, the communal fasting was to be held inside an inflatable, one-hundred-by-one-hundred-foot polyethylene pillow. The structure, dubbed Liferaft Earth, was designed by Charlie Tilford, a graduate student in engineering at Columbia University, and the participants were to live exclusively within it for the duration of the fast. But the organizers could neither secure a prominent site nor

a permit for the innovative shell, which was deemed to be a fire risk, and so the event took place instead in a motel parking lot in the city of Hayward. There, a four-foot-high inflatable wall delineated a compound within which those who were fasting camped. The press and the curious lingered outside the wall, joined by the occasional participant who could no longer bear the hunger pangs, made worse by the temptations of a nearby Chinese restaurant.

Symbolically, the raft also offered refuge for planet Earth. A photograph in the *Whole Earth Catalog* from January 1970 shows an inflated globe among the spread-out paraphernalia of the counter-cultural gathering, thus making the hunger show one of the earliest events where such a globe became part of the iconography of American environmentalism. (The globe can be seen in Robert Frank's 1969 film of the event, *Liferaft Earth*; by the end, it was sadly deflated and abandoned, after inclement weather had made the group decide to relocate to the Portola Institute in Menlo Park.) Today, barely an Earth Day celebration takes place during which the participants do not pass an inflatable globe over their heads in order to express a symbolically

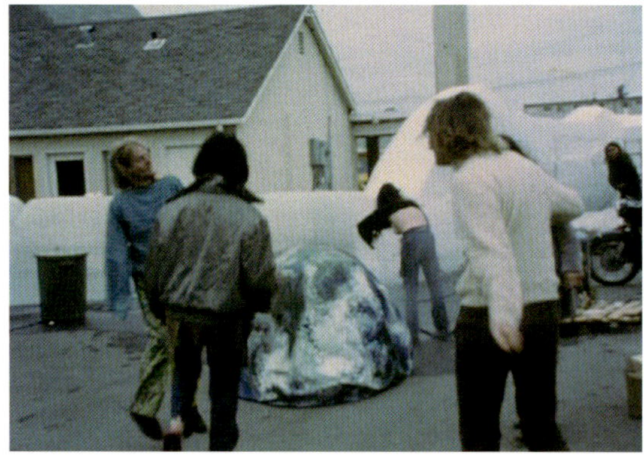

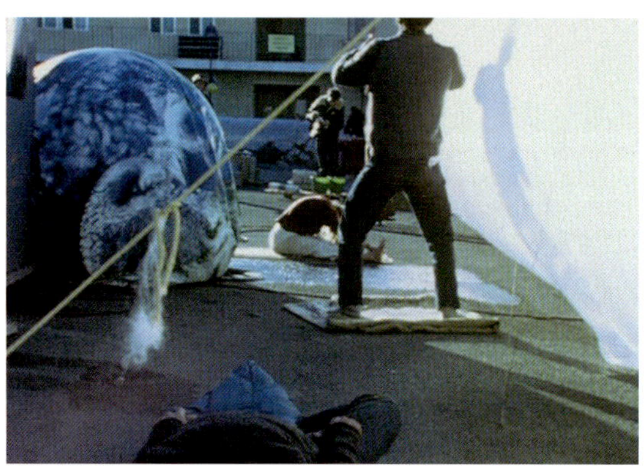

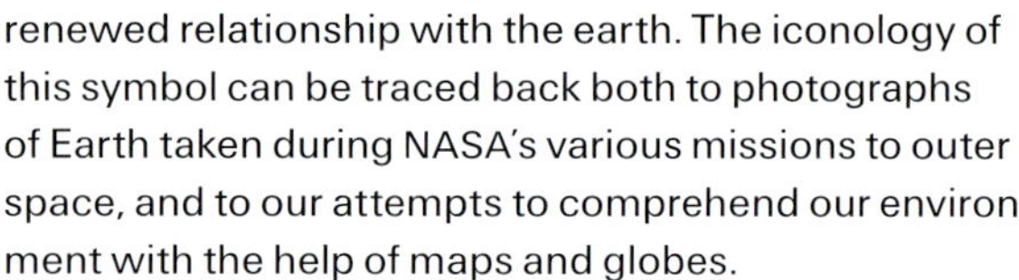

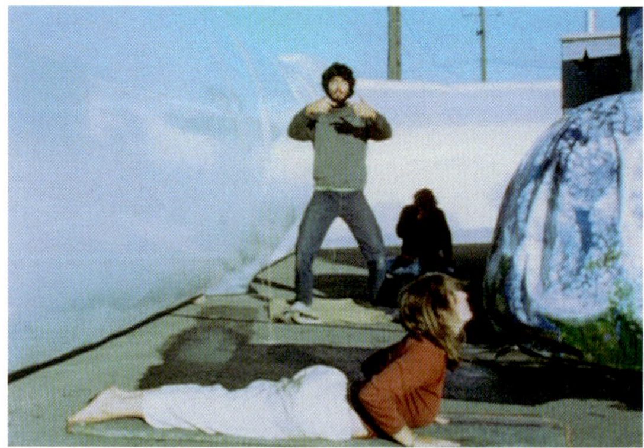

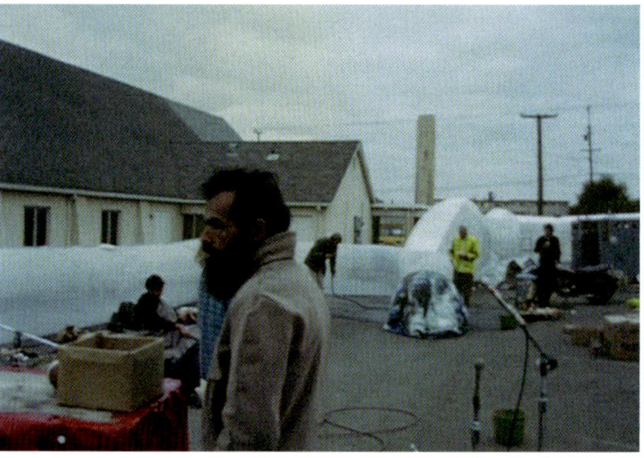

renewed relationship with the earth. The iconology of this symbol can be traced back both to photographs of Earth taken during NASA's various missions to outer space, and to our attempts to comprehend our environment with the help of maps and globes.

. . .

With the advent of space flight in the mid-twentieth century, man's gaze paradoxically turned back toward the earth. The story has often been told of how the astronauts of the *Apollo 8* mission in 1968 snapped, almost accidentally, photographs of their home planet when approaching it from behind the moon.[1] From that point on, images like the famous *Blue Marble*, shot on 2 December 1972 during the *Apollo 17* flight, lent legitimacy to both the space program and twentieth-century concerns for Earth's ecosystems.

On the one hand, pictures of Earth floating in outer space proved the viability of leaving the planet to explore the unknown. Considered from that perspective, the backwards glance was simply the last view of the home planet of an otherwise forward-looking human race—a gaze comparable, perhaps, to the fixed stare at the disappearing cliffs of England of the couple at the center of Ford Madox Brown's 1855 painting *The Last*

of England. On the other hand, the same images took on a near sacred aura for those who, like the advocates of the Whole Earth movement, were searching in the later 1960s for a new relationship between mankind and Mother Earth. To them, the images showed the vulnerability of a planet that appeared fragile and lonely amid the blackness of outer space.

Chronologically, however, inflatable earth balls preceded such imagery, and became the first symbol that 1960s environmentalism adopted in order to act out a new existential relationship with the earth. While playing with an inflatable globe seemingly promoted this emerging sensibility, the motif—man playing with the earth—in fact recalls earlier images from the history of modernity's relationship to the planet.

Globes are one way of representing the earth. Initially of rather small size, large-scale spheres from the nineteenth century onwards allowed for more direct forms of encounter. For example, in 1851 the map publisher James Wyld erected in London a wooden sphere sixty feet in diameter that could be entered

above: Stills from Robert Frank's film *Liferaft Earth*, 1969. The film, which was made at the request of Stewart Brand to document the hunger show protest in Hayward, California, shows the large earth ball around which protesters danced, practiced yoga, slept, and bathed.

in order to study the world that was painted on the inside. It was followed in 1900 by the "Great Globe" conceived—though never realized—by the French anarchist-geographer Elisée Reclus and the architect Louis Bonnier for the World Exposition in Paris, and, fast-forwarding to the mid-twentieth century, by various globes proposed by Buckminster Fuller. In 1956, Fuller envisioned a "Minni Earth" in front of the United Nations in New York as a visual reminder of the immense scope of the organization's global tasks. By the early 1960s, Fuller and his then-colleague John McHale from the British Independent Group had further reduced the globe to a "Miniature Earth," a geodesic sphere covered with a textile skin upon which the silhouettes of the continents were printed. They also developed a geoscope, a small globe into which a man could insert his upper torso in order to view, through sheets of transparent plastic, flickering lights indicating world data such as the distribution of resources: "Viewing the stars through the semi-transparent land masses, from the centre of such a miniature-earth would powerfully locate man in his universe."[2] The diminutive size of the device emphasized man's central position even more than Wyld's globe, as it allowed only one individual at a time to be the center of the world.

Insofar as they too adopt a bird's eye view, aerial and outer-space photographs can be considered an extension of maps. Yet all three differ in regard to their ontological implications for man's relationship with Earth. Some postmodern critiques notwithstanding, maps did aim at understanding the spaces they depicted. Maps not only made these previously uncharted terrains available to explorers, adventurers, and armchair travelers, but, crucially, their initial creation often relied on someone physically traversing the spaces that were subsequently represented (thus the white blotches on early modern Western maps of continents that had not yet been crossed in their entirety by a note-taking explorer). Maps also invite some minor, but conceptually important, physical activity on the part of their readers, who could unlock the abstractly presented physical space by conducting what in German are called *Fingerreisen*: imaginary journeys that take place by moving one's finger from one place name to the next. Earth photographs do not entice similar sensuous engagement with abstract knowledge.

Just over one hundred years passed between the first camera image of a section of the earth, photographed by Nadar from a balloon in 1858, and the extraterrestrial views of segments of our planet taken by the US satellite *Explorer VI* in August 1959.[3] In

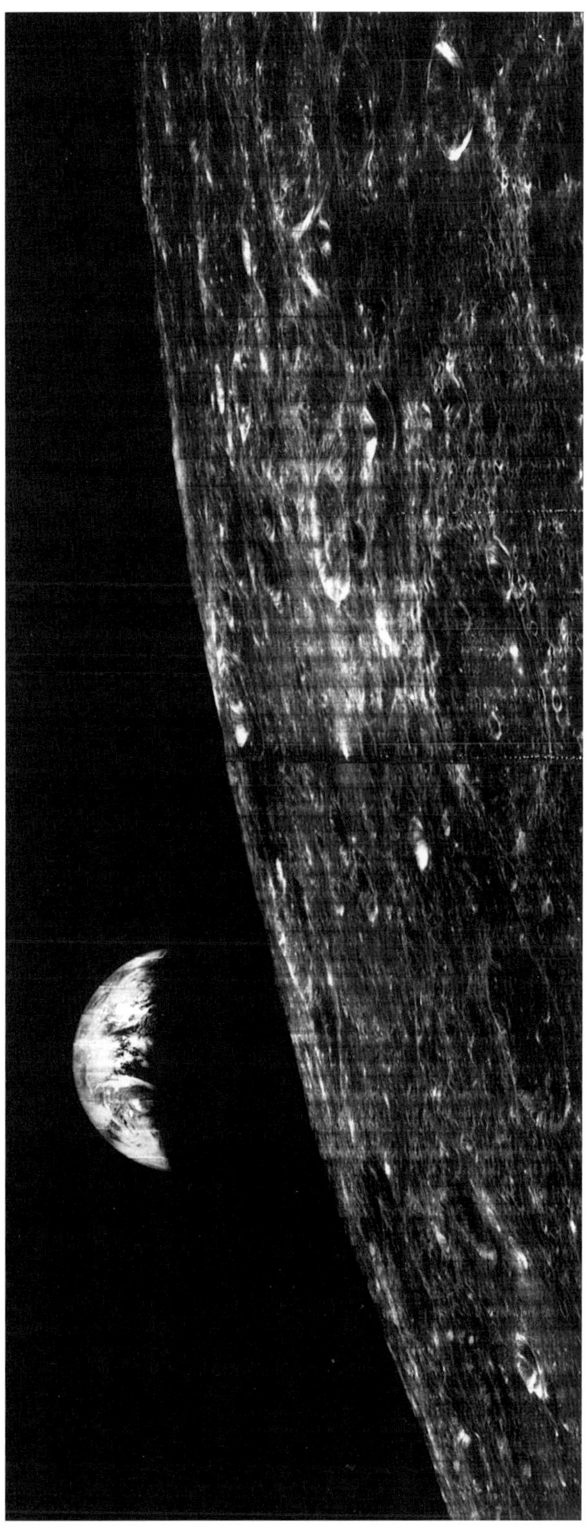

The first ever photograph of an "earthrise" (25 August 1966, *Lunar Orbiter I*). When published by the *New York Times* the next day, the newspaper remarked, "Horizontal orientation lines were added to the picture after it was received by a tracking station near Madrid."

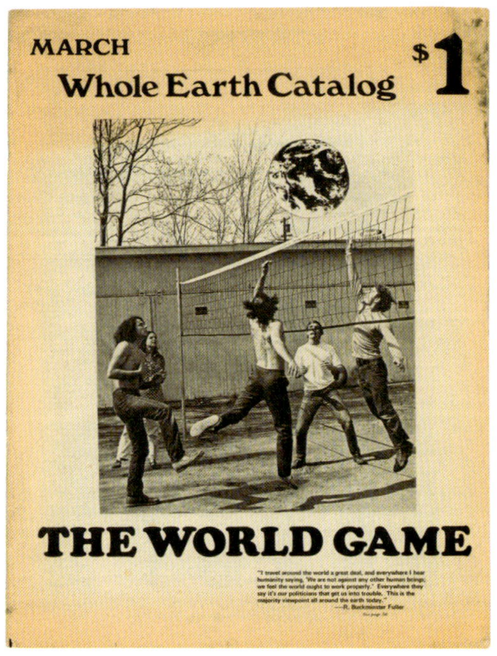

Cover of the *Whole Earth Catalog*, March 1970, illustrated with a collage showing the editorial team enjoying a volleyball game with an earth ball. Courtesy Canadian Centre for Architecture.

between, hot air balloons offered views of Paris, reconnaissance kites allowed for glimpses into enemy trenches during the Great War, and in World War II airplanes achieved the same. In the postwar period, architect Erwin A. Gutkind argued for regional planning on the basis of military aerial photographs that made visible the land between Boston and New York. These images are among the earliest examples of partial earth views buttressing environmentalist thought; Gutkind's essay opened the published proceedings of the 1955 conference "Man's Role in Changing the Face of the Earth" at which the ecological achievements of past and present world civilizations were discussed.

The instant visual overview that photographs of the earth offer suggests usefulness comparable to that of maps. Yet, in the words of art-historian-turned-geographer Denis Cosgrove, though "intensely *geographical*" such images are not, therefore, "cartographic image[s]" —while maps represent in an abstract manner, high-altitude aerial and extraterrestrial photographs offer a more direct, if unusual, depiction of reality. [4] Moreover, these two kinds of photographs themselves differ with regard to scale and the sophistication of the technical equipment used, a difference that marks a fundamental change in man's relationship with planet Earth.

Already in the 1880s, the British painter Philip Gilbert Hamerton distinguished landscape paintings from

bird's eye views by pointing to a qualitative shift from the world as "men see it who dwell in it, and cultivate it, and love it" to the "world as the angels may see it from the midst of space." [5] The increasing ability of later twentieth-century man to view the earth from ever further away in outer space constitutes another qualitative shift, this time from viewing parts of the planet to seeing the whole. Looking at a segment of the globe from above mimics the traditional angle of vision of the human eye; almost irrespective of the height, the view remains connected to the viewing subject which, in turn, stays tied to the earth as the object of the glance. Gazing at the entire globe from outer space no longer means looking down, but back from a distance. The height of the former viewpoint is measurable with regards to a base, usually the surface of the planet; the act of measuring establishes, together with gravity, a clear sense of above and below. The loss of this grounded dimension in gravity-free outer space means that height morphs into mere distance between objects, such as spaceships full of astronauts and planets like the earth. Consequently, outer-space travel initiated, according to philosopher Günther Anders, a process of "spatial distancing from the earth" that gradually revealed our planet as "an ownerless celestial body, the flotsam of the universe," while accompanying outer-space photographs illustrated man's "cosmic eccentricity" as an accidental bystander somewhere in space. [6]

Until outer-space photography truly took off in 1946, when a US program affixed cameras to captured German V2 rockets, extraterrestrial depictions of the earth relied on human imagination and interpolations from existing knowledge. In 1885 Hamerton envisioned the final leg of Archangel Raphael's journey from Heaven to Earth with the words, "At last, when we come within ... twenty thousand miles, we should distinguish the white icy poles, the vast blue oceans, the continents and larger islands glistening like gold in the sunshine, and the silver-bright wandering fields of cloud." [7] Not surprisingly, British astrophysicist Fred Hoyle arrived at a similar impression when he anticipated, during a 1949 BBC radio lecture, the coming of a whole earth picture: "There will be all shades of

---

opposite: New Games Festival, Perkasie, Pennsylvania, 1980. The New Games Foundation sold this type of ball (which had a canvas exterior and heavy-duty vinyl bladder interior) with only the continents outlined, so that the image of the earth's surface had to be painted by hand. The game being played here is called Orbit. Participants would form a circle, with one player in the center, all holding the earth ball aloft. The center participant would try to push the ball outside of the circumference of the circle, while those on the edges would try to keep it within the circle. As with all New Games, there was no scoring system or competitive goal to Orbit. Photo Lee Rush.

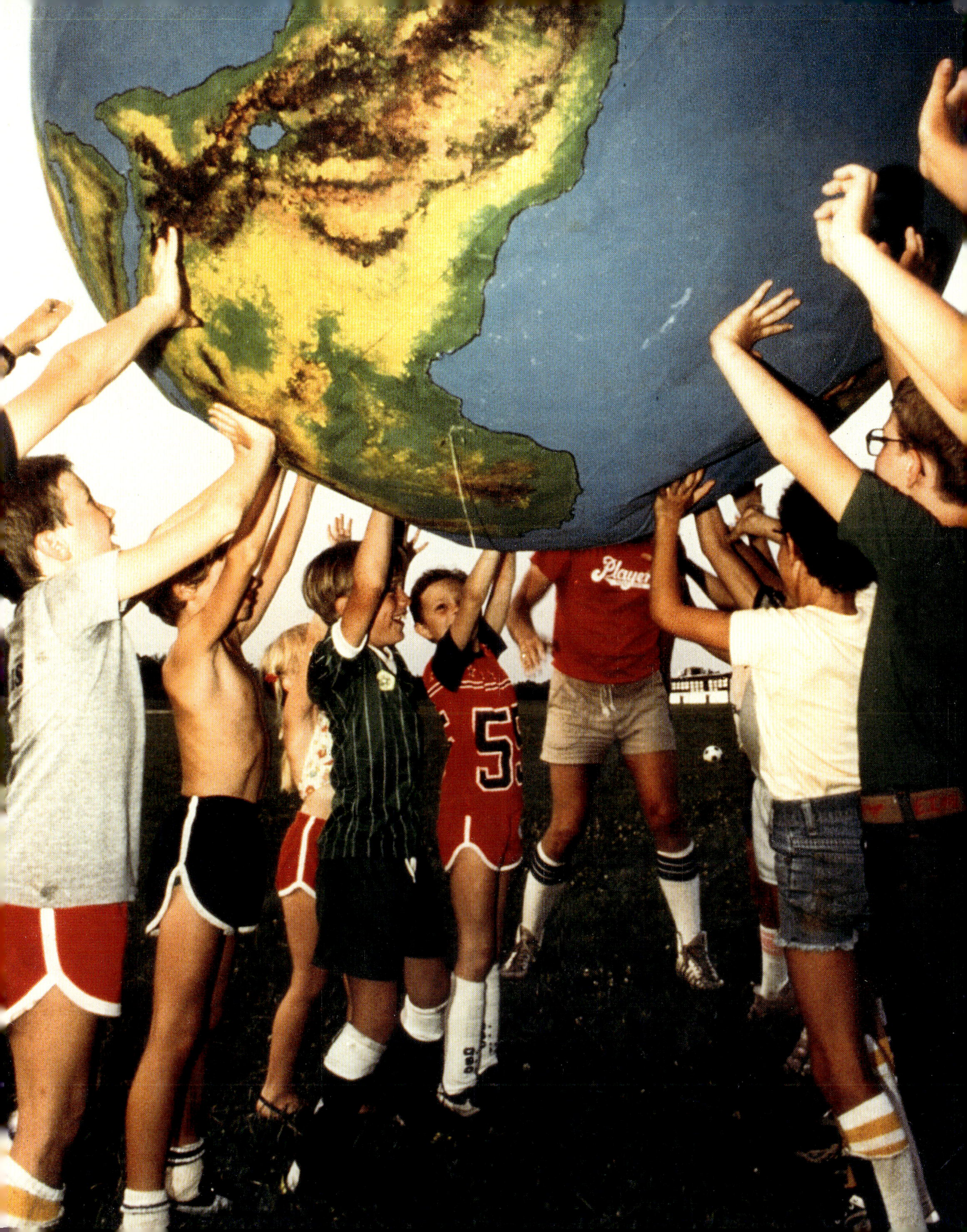

green, varying from the light green of young crops to the sombre darkness of the great northern forests. The desert will show as dusky red, and the oceans will appear as huge areas that look grimly black."[8]

At the time of Hoyle's lecture, the American V2 program had already delivered the first outer space images from sixty-five miles up. Technology progressed rapidly. In 1959, rockets reached seven hundred miles and *Explorer VI* offered an early, more permanent base in outer space for taking photographs. Other satellites followed in quick succession until, in August 1966, *Lunar Orbiter I* sent an image showing the earth partially covered with a semi-circular shadow thrown by the moon.[9] Contrary to Hoyle's claim that "the whole spectacle of the Earth would very likely appear ... as more magnificent than any of the other planets,"[10] the earliest photographs were not all that impressive. They showed semi-circular or near-circular shapes set against streaky black and white backgrounds.[11]

Nevertheless, newspapers welcomed every new image as a "first" with regard to distance from Earth, technical equipment used, and size of surface captured. The V2 pictures from 1946 were followed a year later by the first picture from the landmark a altitude of one hundred miles. The "First Television Picture of the Earth from Space" was broadcast in 1959; 1966 saw both the "First Picture [that] shows Cover of Clouds," and the first picture of the *full* earth, courtesy of the *ATS 1* satellite, one free of any shadow cast by the moon and therefore resembling a *circle* or *disc* (as opposed to the *sphere* of the *whole* earth).[12] Thereafter, things turned colorful with the US Navy's *DODGE* satellite supplying a color picture on 25 July 1967, and NASA's first following on November 16.[13] This series of "firsts" recalls Anders's interpretation of the way in which every forthcoming space flight during the 1960s was anticipated as "historic." The inflationary use of the adjective did not retrospectively identify truly influential past events. Instead, it reduced the "historic" to a present that was instantaneously superseded by the next occurrence.[14] Comparably, to call every new Earth image "first" transformed awesome technological achievements into fleeting moments; almost as soon as they were shot, extraordinary images became ordinary by being drawn into the realm of the everyday.

Moreover, until photographs of the entire earth were technically achievable, the limited field of view available from lower altitudes meant that the frame of the photograph dissected the planet into random pieces. Even if Earth's curvature was visible in an individual image, little conveyed that these sections were parts of a larger celestial body with defined geometrical limits or even with limitations concerning, for example, its ability to support human life. To arrive at the second viewpoint required a neo-Malthusian gaze that recognized the geometrical circumferences as expressions of the planet's limited resources; this became the popular view of the Whole Earth ideology from the later 1960s onwards.

As Stewart Brand began to ponder in early 1966 the ideas that eventually crystallized in the *Whole Earth Catalog*, he started selling little white buttons that asked: "Why haven't we seen a photograph of the Whole Earth yet?" Crucial is the adjective *whole*, as Brand explained in a later essay, for "the earth [is] curved ... closed on itself."[15] This fact, while knowable in the abstract, had not up until then been visible to the inhabitants of the planet; thus, he continued, "people perceived the earth as flat and infinite, and that ... was the root of all their misbehavior." Changing such erroneous perception required the holistic expansion of man's consciousness, to fully grasp "that it [Earth] was curved, think it, and finally feel it." Subsequently, Brand conceived "a six-foot diameter canvas and rubber pushball of the type he had played with in Army boot-camp training. This one [was] painted with continents, oceans, and cloud swirls."[16] This first "earth ball" was created in 1966 for the New Games, an initiative that aimed at channeling human aggression into non-competitive and peaceful tournaments. In short, two years before an image of the entire earth was featured in 1968 on the cover of the *Whole Earth Catalog*'s inaugural issue, Whole Earth environmentalism had already adopted as its symbol an inflatable globe that mimicked the earth as seen from outer space rather than being a three-dimensional model of a two-dimensional world map.

Inflatable earth balls also addressed a major visual drawback of the 1966, first-ever photograph of the full earth, namely, its flat, disc-like appearance—a rather unfortunate result given that man's long quest for outer space travel had begun with the realization that the earth was not the flat center of the universe. While photographs of flat discs did not nourish a sensuous encounter between man and Earth, cuddly inflatable earth balls almost instinctively did. Games with the rubber sphere started by collectively "donating one's breath" to the earth.[17] Having thus taken possession of the planet by inflating it, earth balls were thrown around, rolled up and down hills, and had to endure hirsute hippies throwing themselves at and over them as everyone welcomed "the chance to play with the planet, whether ... pushing, passing or throwing it;

kicking or hugging it; on top, beneath, or against it."[18] This may have been a joyful and novel interaction, but the ease with which the earth was turned into a toy firmly roots this motif in modernity.

In antiquity, Atlas could barely move, so heavy weighed the planet on his shoulders and so tight was the link between man and Earth. Modernity gradually took that weight off man until space travel tore apart his final ties to Earth by offering what Anders called an "opportunity for abstraction," the latter word derived from the Latin word for "to tear away from."[19] Along the path toward the ultimate extraterrestrial step, man had often dreamed of playing, for good or ill, with his planet. In Grandville's *Juggler of Universes* (1844), a clown casually tosses planets, an early warning not to interfere with either the natural course of the universe or the earthly order of things; Charlie Chaplin's *Great Dictator* (1940), in which the despot twirls the globe on his finger tip, warned about a different, deadly presumptuousness, in this case that of 1930s Germanic man. Despite all these warnings and apprehensions, during the 1960s and 1970s earth balls were nonchalantly kicked across New Games fields and hit over volleyball nets.

Considering that extraterrestrial travel had catapulted man into spatial dimensions so vast as to be unfathomable, this reaction may astonish. Yet, one response to the expansion of human experience, argues Anders, was to reign in the newly accessible universe by drawing it back into an orbit that was solely defined by the scale of the human mind and body. Accordingly, for some, accepting this new dimension of human life meant merely determining the best place for the box through which the universe would enter their homes in the form of TV signals: "To the right the record rack, to the left the house bar, and in the centre, the universe hovers as a third piece of furnishing."[20] This focus on human spatiality is why it was not the *Lunar Orbiter I* photograph of the whole earth published in 1966[21] but instead a near-identical one, taken two years later from *Apollo 8*, that acquired fame as the iconic "earthrise" image. This was, first of all, because it was astronauts, and not a satellite, who took the photograph; more importantly, however, the earthrise image was at some point flipped ninety degrees, a move that shifted the moon from its upright position at the right edge of the frame to a horizontal one that grounded man again in relation to a recognizable horizon.[22]

Others, for example members of the counterculture, tried to grasp this new universe through a parallel expansion of human consciousness. By tossing around the earth in the form of an inflatable ball, they symbolically adopted outer space as their newest playground. And yet, as their own literature makes clear, they never managed either to escape Earth's field of gravity or to counter mainstream culture. Instead they simply rehearsed well-established modernist tropes: playing with the globe, as a New Games movement leader, Andrew Fluegelman, asserts, should be understood as nothing more than "a basic human drive for ascension, or simply the wish to be 'sitting on top of the world.'"[23]

The research for this article was supported by the Canadian Centre for Architecture, Montreal, where I was privileged to be a scholar in residence during the summer of 2009.

1 For example: Denis Cosgrove, "Contested Global Visions: *One World, Whole Earth*, and the Apollo Space Photographs," *Annals of the Association of American Geographers*, vol. 84, no. 2 (June 1994), pp. 270–294; and Robert Poole, *Earthrise: How Man First Saw the Earth* (New Haven: Yale University Press, 2008).
2 John McHale, "The Geoscope," offprint of article, no source given, no date, no page. Available in the archives of the Canadian Centre for Architecture, Montreal (BIB 194082).
3 See <grin.hq.nasa.gov/abstracts/gpn-2002-000200.html>. Accessed 14 September 2010.
4 Denis Cosgrove, op. cit., p. 275.
5 Philip Gilbert Hamerton, *Landscape* (London: Seeley & Co., 1885), pp. 3–4.
6 Günther Anders, *Der Blick vom Mond: Reflexionen über Weltraumflüge* (Munich: C. H. Beck, 1970), pp. 66, 59, 60. All translations by the author.
7 Philip Gilbert Hamerton, op. cit., p. 3.
8 Fred Hoyle, *The Nature of the Universe: A Series of Broadcast Lectures* (Oxford: Basil Blackwell, 1950), pp. 9–10.
9 *New York Times*, 26 August 1966. See also <grin.hq.nasa.gov/abstracts/GPN-2000-001588.html>. Accessed 14 September 2010.
10 Fred Hoyle, op. cit., p. 10.
11 See for example <grin.hq.nasa.gov/abstracts/gpn-2002-000200.html> for an image taken from *Explorer VI* on 14 August 1959. Accessed 15 September 2010.
12 *The Chicago Daily Tribune*, 21 November 1946; *The New York Times*, 21 March 1947; *The New York Times*, 29 September 1959; *The New York Times*, 26 August 1966.
13 Beaumont Newhall, *Airborne Camera: The World from the Air and Outer Space* (New York: Hastings House, 1969), pp. 118–121.
14 Günther Anders, op. cit., pp. 68–70.
15 Stewart Brand, "Why Haven't We Seen the Whole Earth?" in Lynda Rosen Obst, *The Sixties: The Decade Remembered Now, by the People Who Lived It Then* (New York: Random House, 1977), p. 168. Italics in the original.
16 Andrew Fluegelman, ed., *The New Games Book: Play Hard, Play Fair, Nobody Hurt* (Garden City, NY: Headlands Press, 1976), p. 9.
17 Ibid.
18 Ibid., p. 143.
19 Günther Anders, op. cit., p. 66.
20 Ibid.
21 *The New York Times*, 26 August 1966.
22 Compare the version of NASA image 68-HC-870 <grin.hq.nasa.gov/images/small/gpn-2001-000009.jpg> with the one at <images.jsc.nasa.gov/lores/AS08-14-2383.jpg>. Both accessed 14 September 2010.
23 Andrew Fluegelman, op. cit., p. 67.

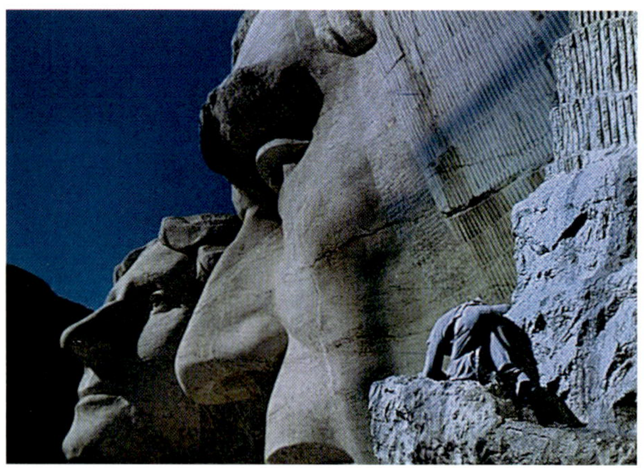

Still from Alfred Hitchcock's *North by Northwest*, 1959.

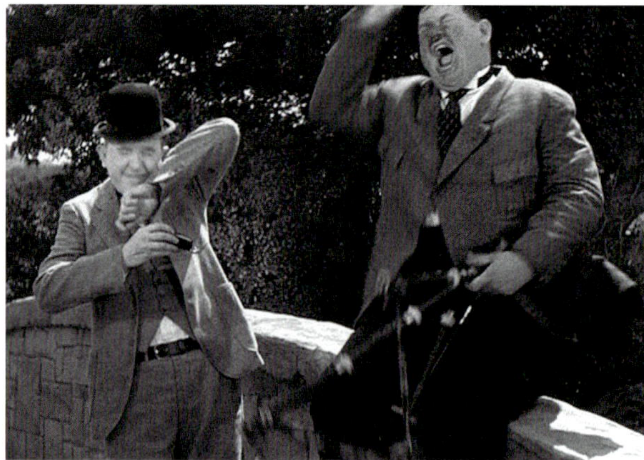

Still from Laurel and Hardy's *Bonnie Scotland*, 1935.

THE CINEMATIC SPASM
AARON SCHUSTER

Rub your hands thrice across your foreheads—
blow your noses—cleanse your emunctories—
sneeze, my good people!
—Laurence Sterne, *Tristram Shandy*

HITCHCOCK'S MISSING SNEEZE

Alfred Hitchcock in conversation with François Truffaut: "I made *North by Northwest* with tongue in cheek; to me it was one big joke. When Cary Grant was on Mount Rushmore, I would have liked to put him inside Lincoln's nostril and let him have a sneezing fit."[1] Imagine Cary Grant, pursued by James Mason's goons, sliding down the presidential proboscis, then hiding in the gaping nostril; or else, suddenly finding himself beneath the massive granite protuberance and pausing to catch his breath. Either way, the gambit is blown by an untimely bout of sneezing. This exquisite nose gag, however, was never filmed. As screenwriter Ernest Lehman recounts: "The Parks Commission was rather upset at this thought. I argued until one of their number asked me how I would like it if they had Lincoln play the scene in Cary Grant's nose. I saw their point at once."

Hitchcock was essentially a comic filmmaker. During a 1967 interview, when asked by an audience member why he'd never made a comedy, the director countered, "But every film I make is a comedy."[2] Along these lines, I believe it is one of Hitchcock's minor films that provides the key to his oeuvre. *The Trouble with Harry*, a film about the upheavals caused in a tranquil rural community by the appearance of an inconvenient corpse, exemplifies two of the defining elements of Hitchcock's cinematic technique: the art of dialectical reversal—the bucolic countryside as the setting for a murder mystery or, in other films, Hitchcock's penchant for cold blondes who signify fiery sexual passion—and the eminently English capacity for understatement, as when the lady who stops a man dragging a corpse ask matter-of-factly, "What seems to be the trouble?" Even *Vertigo*, a cinematic version of Freud's "Mourning and Melancholia" if there ever was one, contains plenty of humorous touches. Think of the droll exchange near the beginning about a brassiere designed by an "aircraft engineer" on the principle of the cantilever bridge—no doubt a reference to the amply bosomed Kim Novak, who replaced the more modestly chested Vera Miles, Hitchcock's first pick for the role of Madeleine/Judy.[3]

Did the master of suspense have a favorite comic scene? In the same interview we read: "I think one of the funniest films I have ever seen is Laurel and Hardy in a film called *Bonnie Scotland*. The longest take I have ever seen on the screen comes when the two of them are standing on a Scottish bridge and Laurel is taking snuff. And he sneezes right into the snuff box. And all the snuff goes into Hardy's face. It was then the longest take I have ever seen before anything happens. And finally, this long sneeze comes. The sneeze is so big that he tilts backwards into the river below. Laurel is left on the bridge and nothing came up but water and fish every few seconds." Perhaps it was this delightful slapstick sequence, with its impeccable timing and exaggerated gestures—Laurel, still on the bridge, is drenched by water launched by Hardy's vigorous sneezes (indeed, at one moment the camera itself is drawn into the whirlpool)—that set Hitchcock's comic imagination into motion. Lehman wanted to write the "Hitchcock picture to end all Hitchcock pictures." What would it mean to film the ultimate sneeze?

This impressive respiratory reflex, which can spew some forty thousand particles at a rate estimated between 90 and 650 miles per hour (nearly eighty-five percent the speed of sound), has long inspired the human imagination and given rise to all kinds of mythic beliefs and speculations. There is a whole "romance and tragedy" of sneezing across cultures and history, a seemingly universal fascination with the explosive bodily phenomenon as remarkable sign, omen from the gods, or vehicle for the soul's passage.[4] And though a marginal topic, it has even on occasion elicited serious philosophical inquiry.[5]

The philosophy of the sneeze can be said to have begun with Aristotle, who in the *History of Animals* wrote that "sneezing is the only sort of breath that has divinatory significance and is supernatural."[6] In the section of *Problems* concerned with the nostrils, the philosopher analyzed questions such as: Why does sneezing stop hiccups? (The violence of the sneeze breaks up the trapped air which causes hiccups); Why does looking at the sun provoke sneezing? (Aristotle attributes what we now call the "photic sneeze reflex"[7] to the heat of the sun evaporating bodily moisture, producing an excess of breath which is then expelled through the nose); Why is sneezing considered divine, but not farting and burping? (The head is the most sacred part of the body); and, Why does man sneeze more than any other animal? (Human beings have a unique combination of wide breath channels and small, short nostrils).

In contrast to this classic systematic approach, Aristotle's teacher presented the sneeze in a much more playful fashion, as a figure of humor and romance in a dramatic scene. Plato's *Symposium*, one of the great texts on love in the Western tradition, is also the site of one of its most profound sneezes, occurring at a crucial turning point in the dialogue.[8] During the speech of Pausanias, Aristophanes suffers from a fit of hiccups, forcing a rearrangement of the order of the speakers (the pure slapstick aspect of the *Symposium* is highly underappreciated—one has to imagine Pausanias lecturing the half-inebriated party guests about Athenian law on pederasty with Aristophanes all the while hiccupping in the background). Eryximachus, a medical doctor (whose name means hiccup- or belch-fighter), takes Aristophanes' place after counseling the comedic playwright on various hiccup cures—hold your breath, gargle with some water, or else tickle your nose with something and sneeze. At the end of his discourse, in which love is portrayed as harmony and proper order,

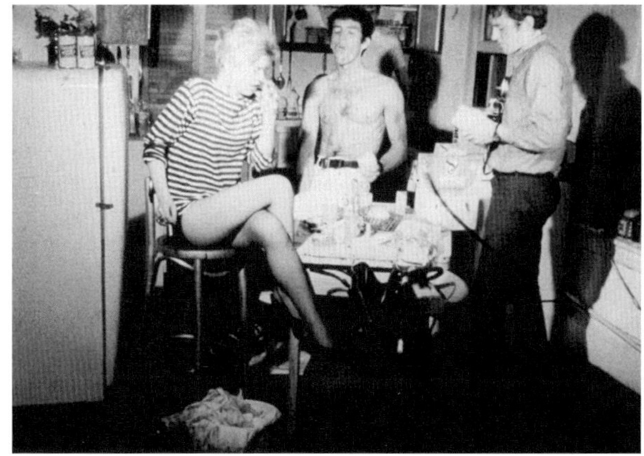

In Andy Warhol's 1965 film *Kitchen*, Edie Sedgwick sneezes every time she forgets her lines and needs to look at parts of the script hidden strategically around the set. Still courtesy Andy Warhol Museum.

the good doctor observes that Aristophanes' hiccups have finally stopped. "Indeed," Aristophanes remarks, "[the hiccupping] did cease, yet not before in fact the sneeze was administered to it, so as to cause me to wonder that the orderly part of the body desires the sort of noises and ticklings of which the sneeze itself consists. For [the hiccupping] ceased just as soon as I administered the sneeze to [the orderly part]."[9] Before launching into his tragic theory of love as the search for the missing half, the hiccuping-sneezing episode allows Aristophanes to open with a quick satire of Eryximachus's medical wisdom: as the sneeze cure would seem to demonstrate, the restoration of order in the body is ironically produced through the combination of two disorders. What else might Plato be telling us if not that, in the case of Eros, only one spasm can "cure" another?

THE MODERN SNEEZE: DUCHAMP AND WARHOL

Plato's playful linkage of the sneeze with Eros has been confirmed in later approaches to the phenomenon. The properly modern, twentieth-century sneeze is best exemplified by a pair of artworks, one by Marcel Duchamp, the other by Andy Warhol, which have some remarkable, if unintended, resonances between them.

Duchamp's assisted readymade, *Why Not Sneeze Rose Sélavy?* (1921), consisting of blocks of marble shaped like sugar cubes, a thermometer, and a cuttlebone shut inside a birdcage, all painted white, is one of the stranger of his constructions, doing for sneezes what his jagged cubist painting did for staircase-descending nudes. "Of course the title seems weird to you," Duchamp remarked, "since there's really no connection between the sugar cubes and a sneeze. First of all there's the dissociational gap between the idea of sneezing and the idea of *Why not sneeze?* because after all, you don't sneeze at will; you usually sneeze in spite of your will. So, the answer to the question, Why not sneeze? is simply that you can't sneeze at will!"[10] If the first part of the title plays on the involuntary nature of the sneeze,[11] the second conjures its erotic quality: Rose Sélavy is a wordplay on *Eros c'est la vie*, "Eros is life," and the pseudonym adopted by Duchamp in the 1920s, which he later spelled Rrose to underline the pun. If Rose/Eros does not sneeze, it is perhaps because, true to her nature as the child of Lack and Craftiness, the final satisfying release is left in abeyance.[12]

But there's more: "And then there's the literary side if I may call it that, but 'literary' is such a stupid word, it doesn't mean anything … but at any rate there's the marble with its coldness, and this meant that you can even say you're cold, because of the marble, and all of the associations are permissible."[13] Like perhaps catching a cold (if I may be allowed this association, which does not, however, work in the original French)? This brings us to Warhol's *Kitchen* (1965), a film meant as a vehicle for Factory superstar Edie Sedgwick, and scripted by Theater of the Ridiculous inventor and key Warhol collaborator Ronald Tavel. *Kitchen* is one of the artist's lesser-known films, and it is still difficult to see a copy today; a year later, Tavel and Warhol would make the more renowned *Chelsea Girls*. Despite its obscurity, *Kitchen* is noteworthy for its aimless witty dialogue and its claustrophobic atmosphere. Norman Mailer enthused that "one hundred years from now they will look at *Kitchen* and see the essence of every boring, dead day one's ever had in a city and say, 'Yes, that is the way it was in the late Fifties, early Sixties in America. That's why they had the war in Vietnam. … That's why the horror came down.' *Kitchen* shows that better than any other work of that time."

Like *Why Not Sneeze Rose Sélavy?*, the movie takes place entirely in its own cramped little "cage": sound- and cameraman Buddy Wirtschafter's wholly white SoHo loft kitchen. The "mollusk-memoried" actress (in the words of Tavel) had trouble learning her lines, so parts of the script were hidden strategically throughout the set, and the starlet was told to sneeze whenever she didn't know the text. This made Sedgwick seem like she had a cold, and her many sneezes ended up providing the film with an unexpected comic dimension, punctuating the half-improvised, disjointed conversations bathed in blasé sexuality and downtown disaffection. Between the suspended sneeze of Rose Sélavy and the flurry of them let loose by the sniffling "It girl" lies the sneeze as object of modern conceptual cool.

Let us now return to Hitchcock: the missing sneeze in "The Man in Lincoln's Nose" (one of the original titles of *North by Northwest*) in fact belongs to a venerable cinematic tradition. The Laurel and Hardy snuff-box gag that so delighted Hitchcock was effectively updated in Woody Allen's 1977 film *Annie Hall*, where Allen's character, Alvy Singer, pokes his nose in a cocaine-filled receptacle at a New York soirée, then sends a pricey plume of white powder into the air with a powerful sneeze. Behind all these nasal convulsions lie the antics of the early short film *That Fatal Sneeze* (1907). Directed by Lewin Fitzhamon for Hepworth and Company— Fitzhamon was a master of the emerging cinematic form, directing about four hundred pictures in his career—this madcap one-reeler is to my knowledge the most sustained filmic treatment of the subject. This time it's neither coke nor snuff that sets off the sneezing hijinks, but that classic nasal irritant, pepper. A middle-aged gentleman pours it liberally over his nephew's plate at supper, triggering a sneezing fit and much malicious laughter. The boy exacts his revenge later that night, sneaking into his uncle's room and sprinkling pepper on his personal effects, including his handkerchief. When the uncle awakes in the morning and gets dressed, he quickly succumbs to a sneezing fit, which precipitates an increasingly zany series of events: a bed is overturned, a vegetable stand knocked down, a policeman thrown to the ground, a house destroyed, an old woman's wig propelled into the air, and so on. Eventually, the sneezing becomes so violent it causes the whole world to shake (early special effects technique: the camera is placed on a rocking board).

The exaggerated explosiveness of the sneeze was also exploited for comic effect by the Marx Brothers. In fact, Harpo's only onscreen "line," occurring in *At The Circus* (1939), is a thunderous "Achoo!" which sends the furniture flying across a cramped little room. But *That Fatal Sneeze* goes one giant sternutation further. At the very end of the film, the poor man literally sneezes himself into oblivion, exploding in a cloud of white smoke—an optical illusion created by stopping the camera and replacing the actor with a small smoke pot. This scene may be viewed as staging a fundamental nasal fantasy: the supreme sneeze is a lethal one. And indeed, there is a long history connecting sneezing with death.

In the Middle Ages, the Bubonic Plague lent an aura of evil to the sneeze; Pope Pelagius II allegedly perished from the disease while sneezing. During the same period, the common practice of blessing a person

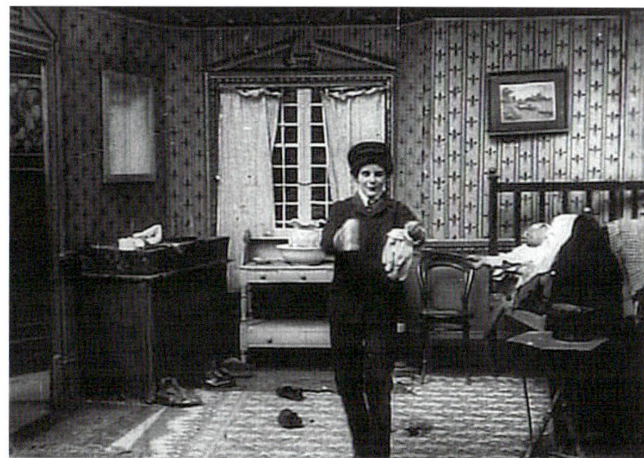

Still from Lewin Fitzhamon's *That Fatal Sneeze*, 1907.

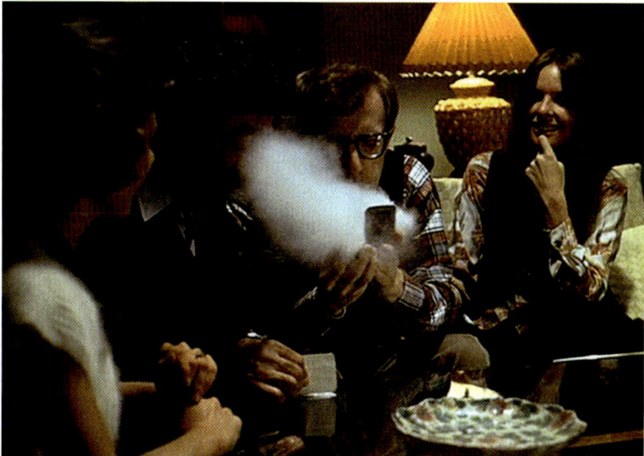

Still from Woody Allen's *Annie Hall*, 1977.

after sneezing gained a new urgency; Pope Gregory VII enjoined his followers to say "May God bless you" as an equivalent to "I hope you may rid yourself of the bacillus."[14] The Greeks considered sneezes to be miraculous signs; in the *Odyssey*, Penelope interprets her son's sneeze as a divine confirmation of her death wish against her suitors. Sneezes without prophetic relevance, on the other hand, were viewed as a disturbance of the gaseous or windy life-soul—the Greek word for soul is etymologically related to the word for blowing—and following a sneeze it was customary to say, "Zeus, save me."[15] The Romans similarly saw sneezing as a potentially dangerous departure of life-spirit from the head, the passing away of what they called *genius*. In the Jewish tradition, there is an old belief that before the time of Jacob, the first man to perish from illness, sneezing was instantly fatal: a strong nasal blast expelled the life force from the body, reversing the movement of divine animation recounted in Genesis 2:7, "God blew into Adam's nostrils the soul of life."

Such was the "surprising" nature of human mortality in ancient times: no sickness, no debility, no warning signs of any kind, just one sneeze and you're done for.

Cinematic interest in this highly charged reflex may be traced back to the very dawn of filmmaking. One of the first copyrighted motion pictures, inspired by Eadweard Muybridge's photographic studies of motion, was in fact a study of a sneeze. Made by W. K. L. Dickson at the Edison Laboratory and composed of eighty-one frames, this filmic "primal scene" features Fred Ott, an Edison employee who had a penchant for practical jokes. The film, titled *Edison Kinetoscopic Record of a Sneeze*, or simply *Fred Ott's Sneeze*, developed a kind of mythical status, in part due to Ott's tireless self-promotion as the world's "first" movie star, with the sneeze footage put forward as the world's "first" movie. Like all origin stories, this one is mired in exaggerations and half-truths, which were eventually debunked by film historian Gordon Hendricks in a short article published in Adolfas and Jonas Mekas's avant-garde journal *Film Culture*. As Hendricks explains, the movie began as the brainchild of Barnet Phillips, a contributor to *Harper's Weekly* who proposed to Thomas Edison to write an article about the new peephole kinetoscope for which the journalist wanted the recording of a sneeze. The publicity-savvy Edison replied that he would be happy to furnish the requested footage. Two months later, after additional prompting by Phillips, Edison asked his assistant Dickson to shoot *Sneeze*. The film was copyrighted on 9 January 1894, not quite the first of its kind, as Dickson had already copyrighted several other short subjects in the previous months. Phillips's article, "Record of a Sneeze," appeared in *Harper's Weekly* on 24 March, accompanied by a reproduction of the entire footage. An excerpt of the article reads: "The Edison kinetoscope gives the entire record of a sneeze from the first taking of a pinch of snuff to the recovery. As seen in this wonderful mechanical device of Mr. Edison's invention, when he exhibits the series of photographs the figure actually sneezes, and the phonograph as an accompanist sounds the precise 'as–shew'. The illusion is so perfect that you involuntarily say, 'Bless you!'" One crucial detail: in the original proposal for the film, the sneezer was meant to be not the ruddy mustachioed Ott but "some nice-looking young person," "a woman." To paraphrase Godard: all you need to make a movie is a girl and a pinch of snuff.

In reference to *Fred Ott's Sneeze*, Mary Ann Doane writes that "contortions of the body and especially its involuntary and violent movement were perceived as particularly cinematic."[16] It is the unique capacity of cinema to capture and break down movement, to reveal the secrets of normally imperceptible transitions and variations, that makes the sneeze such an attractive filmic subject. In his article, Phillips analyzed the roughly two-second gesture ("this curious gamut of a grimace") into ten constituent stages, each one identified with a corresponding frame: priming, nascent sensation, first distortion, expectancy, premeditation, preparation, beatitude, oblivion, explosion, and recovery. This remarkable phenomenology—practically indistinguishable from a description of religious or sexual ecstasy—again highlights the erotic character of the sneeze, and in her study of pornography, Linda Williams claims that the film ought to be situated between "the prehistoric scientific motion studies of Muybridge and the sensationalist later spectacles that were to mark the more advanced stages of primitive cinema and the primitive hard core."[17] In effect, Edison's film is a rudimentary "money shot" that may be seen as part of the then-emerging *scientia sexualis* which aimed at revealing the secrets of bodily pleasure—especially female pleasure—through the use of photography and clinical observation.

A final cinematic reference makes this link between sneezing and feminine *jouissance* explicit in a totally ridiculous way: in a scene from the Steve Martin romantic comedy *The Lonely Guy* (1984), Larry (played by Martin) finally beds his love interest Iris, who confides that she has never had a "you know what." Larry's initial amorous advances produce no effect, until an inadvertent sneeze sends an ecstatic shudder through Iris's body. Capitalizing on this discovery, the hapless lover performs a series of sneezes in order to induce pleasure in the woman, thereby reversing the standard cultural obsession about female simulation. In this case, man has fake sneezes, woman has real orgasms.

1 Alfred Hitchcock and François Truffaut, *Hitchcock/Truffaut* (New York: Simon & Schuster, 1983), p. 102.

2 Alfred Hitchcock, interviewed by Bryan Forbes, the National Film Theatre, 1967, available at <www.bfi.org.uk/features/interviews/hitchcock.html>. Accessed 26 November 2010.

3 It was during the filming of *The Outlaw* in 1941 that famed aviator Howard Hughes, putting his knowledge of aeronautical engineering to good use, invented the underwire push-up bra for his star Jane Russell. Russell's emphasized *décolletage* resulted in *The Outlaw* being kept out of cinemas for three years by Hollywood's Production Code Administration.

4 I refer to Wilson D. Wallis's wonderfully titled study "The Romance and the Tragedy of Sneezing," *The Scientific Monthly*, vol. 9, no. 6 (December 1919).

5 There are also significant literary treatments of the sneeze. In Anton Chekhov's short story "The Death of a Government Clerk," a low-level bureaucrat accidentally sneezes on the back of the neck of a civilian transport general one night at the opera. He spends the rest of the story trying to apologize for involuntarily spattering the general, but his many attempts to excuse himself are coldly rebuffed; the injured party prefers not to even acknowledge the occurrence of the unfortunate episode. In the end, the hero, exhausted and unforgiven, lies down on his couch and expires, as if (to paraphrase the closing line from Kafka's *The Trial*) the shame of the sneeze will eternally outlive him.

6 Aristotle, *Historia Animalium*, trans. A.L. Peck (Cambridge: Loeb Classical Library, 1965), 1.11.492b.

7 Otherwise known as the ACHOO (autosomal dominant compelling helio-ophthalmic outburst) syndrome.

8 Incidentally, Plutarch reports a theory that considered Socrates' *daimon* to be only a sneeze. See Arthur Stanley Pease, "The Omen of Sneezing," *Classical Philology*, vol. 6, no. 4 (Oct 1911), p. 430.

9 Plato, *Symposium*, trans. W. R. M. Lamb (Cambridge: Loeb Classical Library, 1925), 189a. At one point during his commentary on the *Symposium* in his seminar on "Transference" (1960–1961), Jacques Lacan reports Alexandre Kojève telling him that he will never understand the *Symposium* until he can explain why Aristophanes gets the hiccups. He should have added: and sneezes.

10 Jean-Marie Drot, "Jeu d'Échecs avec Marcel Duchamp," unpublished interview for the soundtrack of a film made by ORTF television, 1963. Quoted in Arturo Schwarz, *The Complete Works of Marcel Duchamp* (New York: Delano Greenidge, 1997), p. 487.

11 As a counterpoint, consider the case of comedian Billy Gilbert, famous for his sneeze routines, who worked with Laurel and Hardy in the 1930s and provided the voice for Sneezy in the Disney production of *Snow White and the Seven Dwarfs*: Gilbert was famous for his remarkable ability to sneeze on cue. This seemingly miraculous mastery over the involuntary recalls the story of Guy de Maupassant, who, among his many talents, was reportedly able to make his member rise at will.

12 As Jerrold Seigel writes, "R[r]ose prefers the state of permanent anticipation that is not sneezing to the release of tension the small explosion would bring: because eros is desire, delay is the only state in which it survives undiminished." *The Private Worlds of Marcel Duchamp: Desire, Liberation, and the Self in Modern Culture* (Berkeley: University of California, 1995), p. 171. In the *Symposium*, Plato recounts the myth of Eros's birth from the union of Poros (Craftiness or Resourcefulness) and Penia (Lack).

13 Arturo Schwarz, op. cit., p. 487.

14 See J. J. M. Askenasy, "The History of Sneezing," *Postgraduate Medical Journal*, vol. 66 (1990), p. 549.

15 I draw here, and in what follows, on Richard Broxton Onians, *The Origins of European Thought: About the Body, the Mind, the Soul, the World, Time, and Fate* (Cambridge: Cambridge University, 1951), pp. 103–105, 132, and passim.

16 Mary Ann Doane, *The Emergence of Cinematic Time: Modernity, Contingency, The Archive* (Cambridge, Mass.: Harvard University, 2002), p. 177.

17 Linda Williams, *Hard Core: Power, Pleasure, and the "Frenzy of the Visible"* (Berkeley: University of California, 1989), p. 52. See also Marjorie Garber, *Symptoms of Culture* (London: Penguin, 1998), pp. 221–225.

opposite: Stills from Edison Film Manufacturing Company's *Edison Kinetoscopic Record of a Sneeze*, 1894. The film is one of a series of short films made by W. K. L. Dickson in January 1894 for advertising purposes. The star is Fred Ott, an Edison employee known to his fellow workers in the laboratory for his comic sneezing and other gags. This film was received in the Library of Congress on 9 January 1894 as a copyright deposit from Dickson and is the earliest surviving copyrighted motion picture. Courtesy Library of Congress.

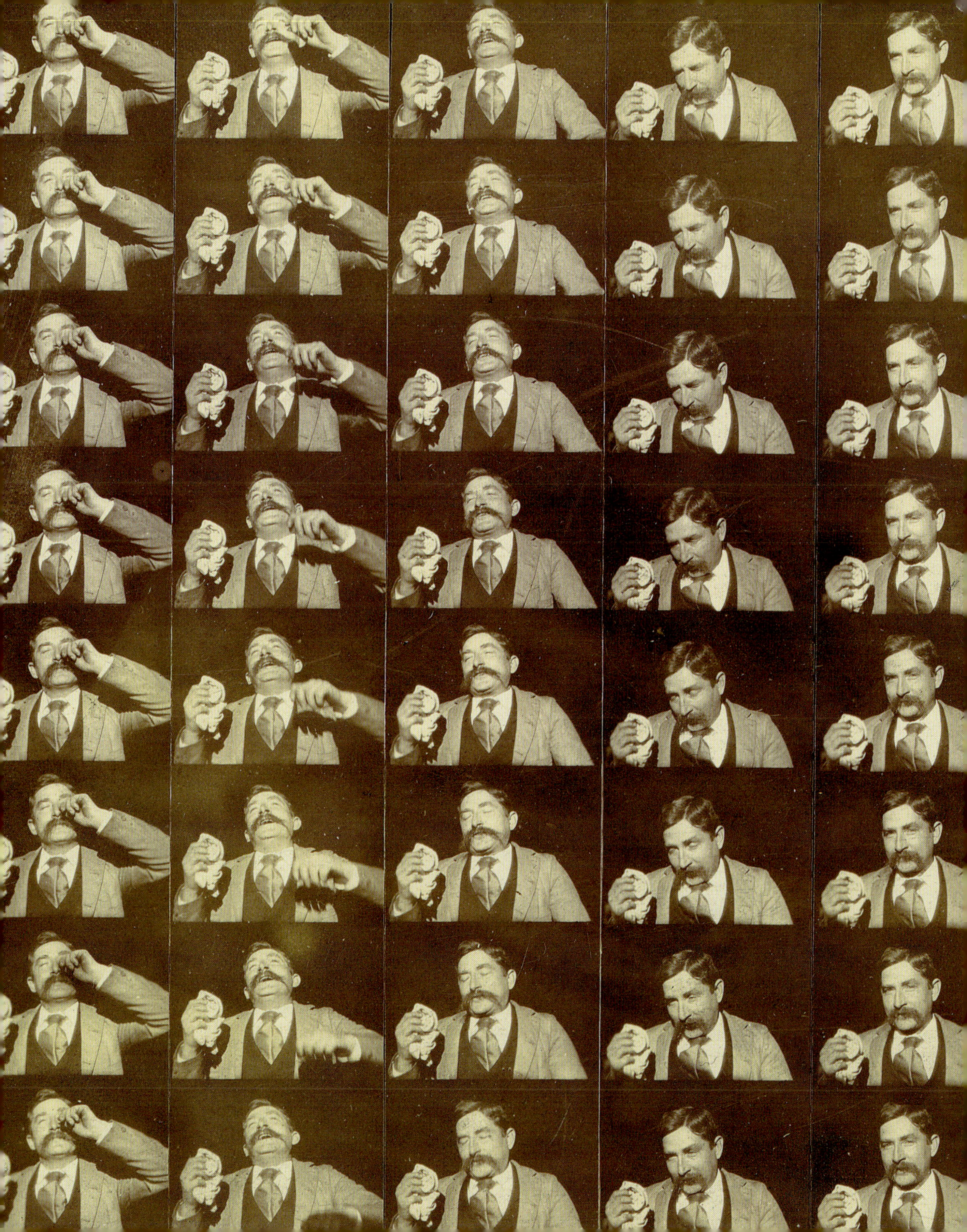

HOW TO MAKE ANYTHING SIGNIFY ANYTHING
WILLIAM H. SHERMAN

For much of his long and largely secret career, Colonel William F. Friedman kept a very special photograph under the glass plate that covered his desk. As desks go, this one saw some impressive action. By the time he retired from the National Security Agency in 1955, Friedman had served for more than thirty years as his government's chief cryptographer, and—as leader of the team that broke the Japanese PURPLE code in World War II, co-inventor of the US Army's best cipher machine, author of the papers that gave the field its mathematical foundations, and coiner of the very term *cryptanalysis*—he had arguably become the most important code-breaker in modern history.[1]

At first glance, the photo looks like a standard-issue keepsake of the kind owned by anyone who has served in the military. Yet Friedman found it so significant that he had a second, larger copy framed for the wall of his study. When he looked at the oblong image, taken in Aurora, Illinois, on a winter's day in 1918, what did Friedman see? He saw seventy-one officers, soon to be sent to the war in France, for whom he had designed a crash course on the theory and practice of cryptology. He saw his younger self at one end of the mysterious group of black-clad civilians seated in the center; and at the other end he saw the formidable figure of George Fabyan, the director of Riverbank Laboratories in nearby Geneva, where Friedman found not just his cryptographic calling but also his wife Elizebeth (flanked here by two other instructors from Riverbank's Department of Ciphers). And he saw a coded message, hiding in plain sight. As a note on the back of the larger print explains, the image is a cryptogram in which people stand in for letters; and thanks to Friedman's careful positioning, they spell out the words "KNOWL-EDGE IS POWER." (Or rather they almost do: for one thing, they were four people short of the number needed to complete the "R.")

The photograph was an enduring reminder, then, of Friedman's favorite axiom—and he was so fond of the phrase that some fifty years later he had it inscribed as the epitaph on his tomb in Arlington National Cemetery.[2] It captures a formative moment in a life spent looking for more than meets the eye, and it remained Friedman's most cherished example of how, using the art and science of codes, it was possible to make anything signify anything. This idea will no doubt strike us as quintessentially modern, if not postmodern, but Friedman took it straight from the great Renaissance scholar-statesman Sir Francis Bacon (1561–1626), along with both the hidden motto in the image and the method used to convey it. In other words, the graduation photo from Friedman's earliest course in military cryptanalysis is at once a tribute to Bacon's philosophy and a master class in the use of his *biliteral cipher*.

Bacon devised this ingenious code in the late 1570s (when he spent three years in the entourage of the English ambassador in France), but he did not describe its workings until 1623.[3] The cipher was based, as the name "biliteral" suggests, on a system using only two letters—or, more precisely, one where each letter in the alphabet is represented by some combination of *a*'s and *b*'s. When Bacon realized that it was possible to represent all twenty-six letters in permutations of only two by using groups of five, he generated the following key:[4]

        A = aaaaa
        B = aaaab
        C = aaaba
        D = aaabb
        E = aabaa
        F = aabab
        G = aabba
        H = aabbb
        I/J = abaaa
        K = abaab
        L = ababa
        M = ababb
        N = abbaa
        O = abbab
        P = abbba
        Q = abbbb
        R = baaaa
        S = baaab
        T = baaba
        U/V = baabb
        W = babaa
        X = babab
        Y = babba
        Z = babbb

The crucial point in Bacon's system is that the *a*'s and *b*'s in the ciphered text are not represented by those actual letters. If they were (using what is known as a straightforward *substitution* cipher[5]), a message reading "Hi" would simply appear as "aabbb abaaa": anyone intercepting the text would quickly see that it was in code, and—given enough text and time—would easily discover the key. His way around this problem was as powerful as it was simple: he allowed the *a*'s and *b*'s in his system to designate the different forms of anything that can be divided into two classes, sorts, or types (which Bacon referred to as the *a-form* and the *b-form*).

If our "infolded" writing (or *plain-text*) is "Hi," we simply need to create an "infolding" text (or *cover-text*) that says anything we want it to but is ten letters long, with the third, fourth, fifth, and seventh letters represented by *b*-types and the rest by *a*-types. These types might, indeed, be typographical, distinguished, say, by bold-face versus regular:

br**ook**ly**n** ny
↓
aabbb abaaa
↓
h i

Or we might toggle between two different fonts (which Bacon called a "bi-formed alphabet"). In the example supplied by Bacon himself, a secret agent is warned to flee through a deceptive cover-text:

Do not go til I come
↓
aabab ababa babba
↓
f l y

The hidden message here is doubly secure because our cover-text can say the opposite of what we mean while looking like plain (if poorly printed) text.[6]

But Bacon added a further twist to the ancient art of *steganography*, the general name for the practice of concealing messages through the use of disguise and deception.[7] In the biliteral cipher, the cover-text need not, in fact, be "text" at all: the *a*'s and *b*'s can be represented by two types of anything—pluses and minuses, flowers of different kinds or colors, even (literally) apples and oranges—and this, for Bacon, is what gives his biliteral system the greatest power of all,

which is to signifie omnia per omina *[anything by means of anything]. ... And by this* Art *a way is opened, whereby a man may express and signifie the intentions of his mind, at any distance of place, by objects which may be presented to the eye, and accommodated to the eare ... as by Bells [and] Trumpets, by Lights and Torches ... and any instruments of like nature.*[8]

When Friedman assembled his students and colleagues in front of the Aurora Hotel to give them a living

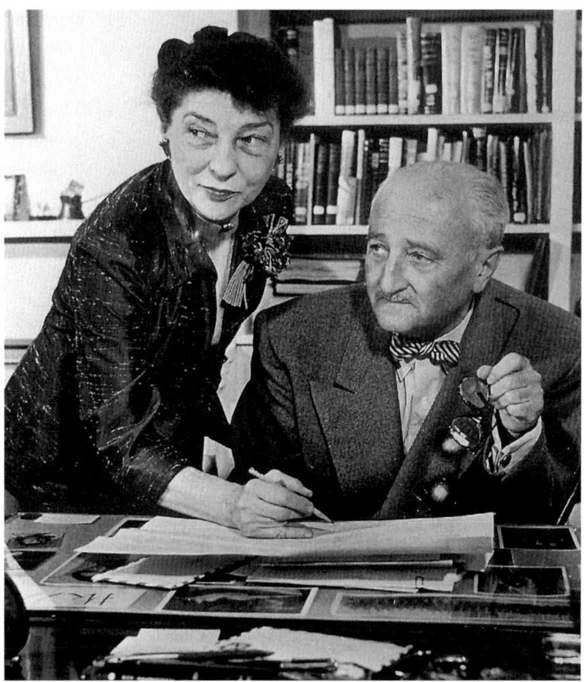

William and Elizebeth Friedman in the study of their Capitol Hill home, ca. 1957. Note the "Knowledge is Power" photograph (included as a poster in this issue) on his desk. Courtesy the George C. Marshall Research Library.

illustration of Bacon's art, he used the most natural instrument of all, their bodies, simply asking the *a*'s to face the camera and the *b*'s to look away. So the seated group of which he was a part would form the sequence "abaab"—which would be a *k* (but not, as it happens, the initial "K" in Bacon's axiom).

It is unlikely that Bacon's cipher system was ever used for the transmission of military secrets, in the seventeenth century or in the twentieth. But for roughly a century from 1850, it set the world of literature on fire. A passion for puzzles, codes, and conspiracies fuelled a widespread suspicion that Shakespeare was not the author of his plays, and professional and amateur scholars of all sorts spent extraordinary amounts of time, energy, and money combing Renaissance texts in search of signatures and other messages that would reveal the true identity of their author. Even after the recent publication of James Shapiro's comprehensive history of the authorship controversy, *Contested Will*, it is difficult for us to appreciate the depth of conviction—among writers as diverse and as distinguished as Mark Twain, Walt Whitman, Sigmund Freud, Henry James, Henry Miller, and even Helen Keller—that Shakespeare's texts contained the secret solution to what was widely considered to be "the Greatest of Literary Problems."[9] Bacon became (for a while) the leading candidate,

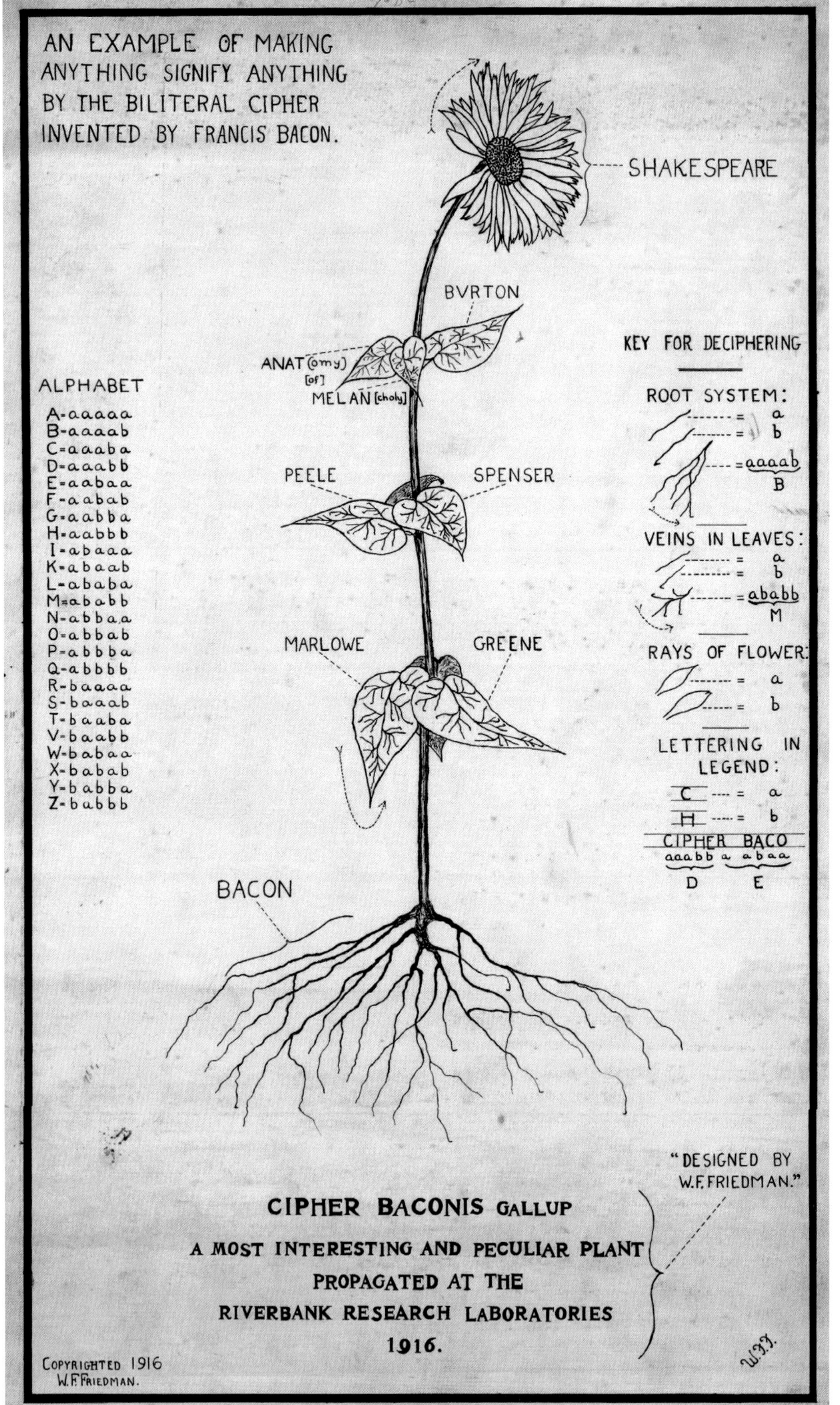

AN EXAMPLE OF MAKING
ANYTHING SIGNIFY ANYTHING
BY THE BILITERAL CIPHER
INVENTED BY FRANCIS BACON.
SHAKESPEARE
BVRTON
ANAT (omy) [of] MELAN [choly]
ALPHABET
A-aaaaa
B-aaaab
C-aaaba
D-aaabb
E-aabaa
F-aabab
G-aabba
H-aabbb
I-abaaa
K-abaab
L-ababa
M-ababb
N-abbaa
O-abbab
P-abbba
Q-abbbb
R-baaaa
S-baaab
T-baaba
V-baabb
W-babaa
X-babab
Y-babba
Z-babbb
PEELE
SPENSER
MARLOWE
GREENE
BACON
KEY FOR DECIPHERING
ROOT SYSTEM:
= a
= b
= aaaab
B
VEINS IN LEAVES:
= a
= b
= ababb
M
RAYS OF FLOWER:
= a
= b
LETTERING IN LEGEND:
C --- = a
H --- = b
CIPHER BACO
aaabb a abaa
D E
"DESIGNED BY W.F.FRIEDMAN."
CIPHER BACONIS GALLUP
A MOST INTERESTING AND PECULIAR PLANT
PROPAGATED AT THE
RIVERBANK RESEARCH LABORATORIES
1916.
COPYRIGHTED 1916
W.F.FRIEDMAN.

and his biliteral cipher—Renaissance England's first and clearest statement about how to hide texts within texts—seemed to offer the "Baconians" (as his champions were known) the key that everyone was looking for.

As late as 1946, the long-running radio program *The New Adventures of Sherlock Holmes* could air an episode called "The Singular Affair of the Baconian Cipher," in which Holmes and Watson set off for Penge in search of "a paralyzed Baconian scholar" who has summoned them with a peculiar piece of printing in their morning newspaper.[10] Friedman's own introduction to the wonderful world of codes had come through Edgar Allan Poe's story "The Gold Bug," which he read as a child, and he later suggested that most people came to cryptography through the genre of detective fiction.[11] But in the early years of the twentieth century, the Baconians thought they had found a truth that was stranger than fiction, and a schoolteacher from Michigan named Elizabeth Wells Gallup inspired a generation of readers to plunge into the plays of Shakespeare with Bacon's biliteral cipher in hand.

Nobody was more excited by Gallup's alleged discoveries than George Fabyan, the eccentric heir to the country's largest cotton-goods firm. Fabyan brought Gallup to his private estate at Riverbank, on the Fox River just west of Chicago. He had the main building redesigned by Frank Lloyd Wright and gradually added a Japanese garden, a Roman-style swimming pool, a working lighthouse, an open-air zoo (with a gorilla named Hamlet), and a Dutch windmill moved brick-by-brick at outrageous expense. Gallup joined an avant-garde faculty of scientists dedicated, as Fabyan put it, to "wresting from Nature, her secrets." Mr. B. E. Eisenour served as dean and director of research in physics, bringing Professor Wallace Sabine from Harvard to continue his pioneering work on architectural acoustics; a Dr. Scott carried out experiments in the medicinal uses of radioactive elements, and a Dr. Henderson worked on hoof-and-mouth disease; and J. A. Powell, former editor of the University of Chicago Press, took up a chair in typography. Gallup was equipped with a team of assistants (including Elizebeth Smith, a young Shakespearean plucked from the stacks of the Newberry Library) and a photographic workroom, where she presided over an "American Academy of Baconian Literature," publishing new work on the biliteral cipher and developing a correspondence course on literary cryptology.

In September 1915, Fabyan lured Friedman away from a PhD in plant biology at Cornell, setting him up as director of the Department of Genetics and putting him to work on the propagation of wheat. But Friedman's interest in photography and bibliography (not to mention Elizebeth Smith) soon brought him into Gallup's Department of Ciphers, where he created many of the images used in Riverbank's Baconian publications. His signature is found in the lower right corner of many of the team's studies of Elizabethan letter-forms, and he seems to have had a hand in most of their "alphabet classifiers," standardized templates designed to be placed over Shakespeare's plays and poems with visual aids to help readers sort the haphazard printing into *a*-types and *b*-types, allowing them to see the messages that Bacon had hidden behind the most famous of all texts. While he would soon lose faith in the methods and the purpose of Gallup's project, Friedman's Baconian initiation was of the utmost importance, both for his personal career and for the development of cryptography as a field.

I have recently stumbled across the archive of Friedman's years at Riverbank (with working notes and manuscript drafts that Friedman himself sought in vain to recover), and it documents his transition from genetics to cryptology and from literary to military codes. It reveals an intuitive grasp of cipher systems that must have been breathtaking: Friedman's instant ability to work—and play—with the biliteral cipher makes his early encounter with Bacon look like Alice's encounter with the looking glass. Sometime in 1916 he designed a card that Gallup and her team used for internal notes and letters to the world beyond Riverbank. It is a botanical drawing of a flower with the witty caption, "CIPHER BACONIS GALLUP / A MOST INTERESTING AND PECULIAR PLANT PROPAGATED AT THE RIVERBANK RESEARCH LABORATORIES / 1916." But Friedman left behind a second version of the image used in teaching, where he reveals that everything on it—including the flower—says something else, using Bacon's now familiar method. He added a new caption at the top, describing it as "An example of making anything signify anything by the biliteral cipher invented by Francis Bacon." The roots of the flower take two forms, bearing the name "Bacon"; the leaves have lines of two types, which yield the names of various Elizabethan authors and books; and the petals can be split into notched and un-notched forms, spelling out "Shakespeare." Even the printed caption at the bottom turns out to be a biliteral cipher, confirming Friedman's authorship of the design (as if there could be any doubt).

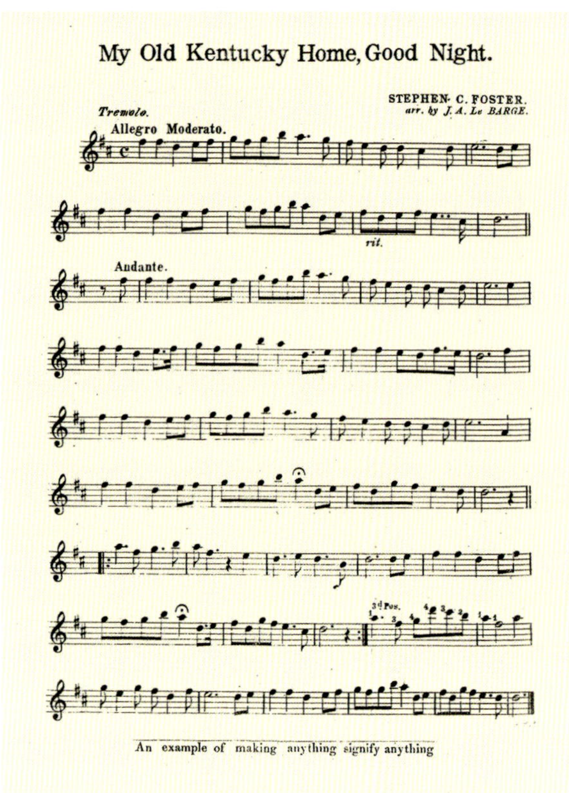

Friedman's coded sheet music. The message reads, "Enemy advancing right / We march at daybreak." Courtesy the New York Public Library.

Another design from the same year used a more innocent cover-text, the sheet music for Stephen Foster's extremely popular nineteenth-century song, "My Old Kentucky Home, Good Night."[12] Only the telltale caption at the bottom, "An example of making anything signify anything," tips us off to the Baconian cipher it contains. This time Friedman left no key, but once we notice that some of the notes have small gaps in them (*b*-types), and some are whole (*a*-types), it does not take long to extract the secret message: "ENEMY ADVANCING RIGHT / WE MARCH AT DAYBREAK."

By the middle of 1917, the enemy was indeed advancing, and it was clear that the US military needed cryptographic expertise of a kind and on a scale that it did not yet have. As the government prepared to enter World War I, it turned to the cryptographic think-tank created by Fabyan and sent a stream of coded correspondence to be broken along with a series of units to be trained. Friedman himself would soon be commissioned

and sent off to France, and while he worked for a few more years at Riverbank after he returned, by the early 1920s he and his wife had moved to Washington for good, where they pursued their long careers with the cryptographic agencies they helped to create. But they kept in close contact with the network of Baconians and in 1954 finished a remarkable study of Gallup and others: it was published in 1957 as *The Shakespearean Ciphers Examined*, and it almost single-handedly put an end to the craze for amateur cryptography in the service of anti-Shakespearean arguments.

But even in that skeptical (and often scathing) book, the Friedmans express their admiration for Bacon's contribution to the field they made their own. Indeed, they remind us of how much the modern world owes to him. Many of the twentieth century's major developments in artistic practice and scientific method derive either from the ability to make anything signify anything or from the problems of mind and meaning this posed. Friedman's early applications of probability to cryptography (like new approaches to psychoanalysis, structural linguistics, literary criticism, and so on) were designed in part to answer the question, "If anything can signify anything, then how do we know what *anything* means?" And in an introductory lecture written in the late 1950s, Friedman finally spelled out the connection between the *a*'s and *b*'s of Bacon's biliteral cipher and the zeros and ones that were creating a new digital age: "Bacon was, in fact, the inventor of the binary code that forms the basis of modern ... computers."[13]

Computers have increased our ability to make anything signify anything in ways that Friedman could not have predicted. A Google search for *steganography* reveals a whole world of digital tools and communities that combine traditional cryptography with cutting-edge computation—and its applications are both more innocent and more sinister than anything produced by the Baconians. Unused bytes and pixels in files can contain huge amounts of invisible information, and by using basic programs and simply changing the settings in a display, a tree can become a cat, a cat can tell us to blow up a bridge, and an oil painting of a whaling expedition can carry the entire text of *Moby Dick*.[14] The codes of the computer age contain more *a*'s and *b*'s than were dreamt of in Bacon's philosophy.

---

1 David Kahn concludes the best account of Friedman's contributions to the field by granting him "the mantle of the greatest cryptologist" of all time; see *The Codebreakers: The Story of Secret Writing* (New York: Macmillan, 1967), p. 393. Ronald Clark's popular biography, *The Man Who Broke PURPLE* (Boston: Little Brown & Co., 1977), offers a useful introduction to Friedman's papers at the

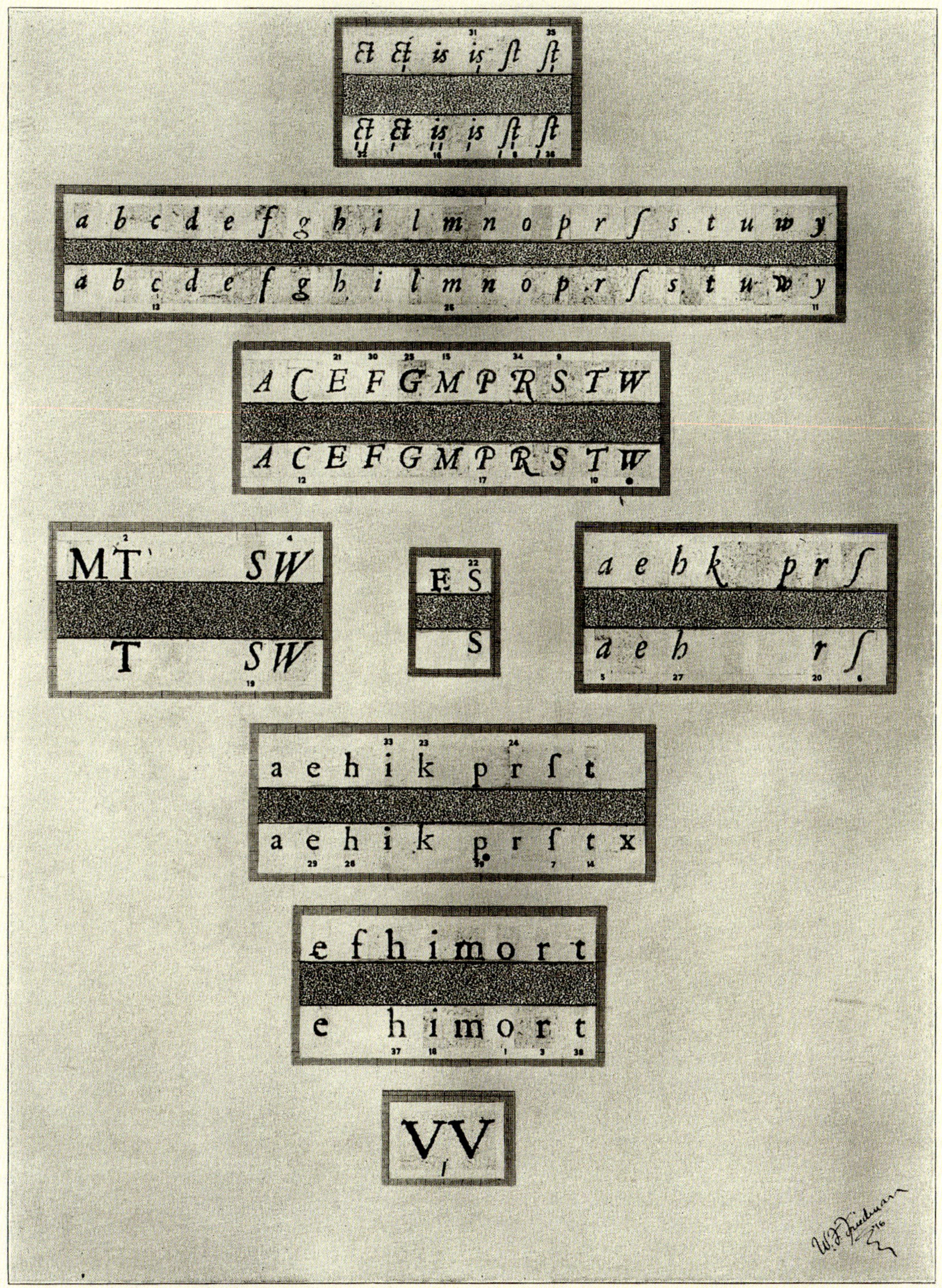

a forms above the shaded parts, b forms below; in the digraph, a stroke indicates the b form

CUT OUT SHADED PART WITH SHARP KNIFE

George C. Marshall Foundation, on the campus of the Virginia Military Institute in Lexington, Virginia. The library's website <www.marshallfoundation.org/library/collection.html> now features a comprehensive guide to the Friedman Collection produced by VMI historian Rose Mary Sheldon, and I am grateful both to Dr. Sheldon and to the staff at the Marshall Foundation—especially Paul Barron and Jeffrey Kozak—for their help and hospitality.

2 See <www.arlingtoncemetery.net/wfried.htm>. Accessed 26 November 2010.

3 Francis Bacon, *De Dignitate & Augmentis Scientiarum*, in *Opera Francisci Baronis de Verulamio* (London: John Haviland, 1623); first translated into English by Gilbert Wats as *Of the Advancement and Proficiencie of Learning* (Oxford: Leonard Lichfield, 1640). The discussion of ciphers is found in book 6, chapter 1. On Bacon's years in France, and his close contact there with "the grand master of intelligence ciphers, Thomas Phelippes," see Lisa Jardine and Alan Stewart, *Hostage to Fortune: The Troubled Life of Francis Bacon,* 1561–1626 (London: Victor Gollancz, 1998), chapter 2.

4 Note that the doubling up of I/J and U/V is not a shortcut: in Bacon's day, they were effectively the same letter, meaning that the English alphabet had only twenty-four letters. Using groups of five yielded thirty-two permutations of *a*'s and *b*'s, more than enough for even the full modern alphabet.

5 In his *Six Lectures on Cryptology*, produced for the National Security Agency in the late 1950s and recently reissued by the NSA's Center for Cryptologic History, Friedman offered the following distinction: "Technically, there are only two distinctly different types of treatment that may be applied to written plain text to convert it into a cipher, yielding two different classes of ciphers. In the first, called *transposition*, the letters of the plain text retain their original identities and merely undergo some change in the relative positions, with the result that the original text becomes unintelligible. ... In the second, called *substitution*, the letters of the plain text retain their original relative positions but are replaced by other letters with different sound values, or by symbols of some sort, so that the original text becomes unintelligible." The Center for Cryptologic History, *The Friedman Legacy* (Fort Meade, MD: National Security Agency, 1992), pp.11–13.

6 I have adapted this example from Bacon's *Of the Advancement and Proficiencie of Learning* (1640), op. cit., pp. 266–268. I have used Univers for *a*'s and Baskerville for *b*'s, but Bacon's original fonts are far closer in style—making the coded text less likely to raise suspicion but also harder to decipher.

7 The practice went back to ancient Greece, but the term was first used in the 1490s by Johannes Trithemius—author of the first printed book on cryptography.

8 *Of the Advancement and Proficiencie of Learning*, op. cit., pp. 265–266. In an earlier discussion of ciphers (from the 1605 first edition of the book), Bacon described "the highest Degree" of ciphering as the ability "to write OMNIA PER OMNIA; which is undoubtedly possible, with a proportion Quintuple at most, of the writing infoulding, to the writing infoulded, and no other restrainte whatsoeuer" (Book 2, fol.61r), but he did not describe his own invention for doing so.

9 James Phinney Baxter, *The Greatest of Literary Problems* (Boston: Houghton Mifflin Co., 1915); James Shapiro, *Contested Will: Who Wrote Shakespeare?* (New York: Simon & Schuster, 2010).

10 This episode was broadcast on 27 May 1946, and it marked Basil Rathbone's final appearance as Sherlock Holmes. The script betrayed more than a passing familiarity with Baconian scholarship: Holmes takes Ignatius Donnelly's *Great Cryptogram* (1888) as common knowledge and offers a casual endorsement of the anti-Stratfordian position.

11 William F. Friedman, "Edgar Allan Poe, Cryptographer," *American Literature*, vol. 8, no. 3 (1936), pp. 266–280. See also Shawn James Rosenheim, *The Cryptographic Imagination: Secret Writing from Edgar Poe to the Internet* (Baltimore: The Johns Hopkins University Press, 1997), chapter 6.

12 The song was first published in 1853 and became the state song of Kentucky in 1928. The version used by Friedman was published in 1903 as part of *The Century Collection of Popular Selections for Mandolin and Guitar.*

13 The Center for Cryptologic History, *The Friedman Legacy*, op. cit., p. 46.

14 See <en.wikipedia.org/wiki/Steganography> and <www.flickr.com/photos/krazydad/257804202>. Both accessed 26 November 2010.

FACING THE UNKNOWN
D. GRAHAM BURNETT

It is a basic problem. Fundamental. Pervasive. The problem at the heart of historical practice, individual identity, collective memory. Art too, perhaps. It is, in effect, the problem of death among the living: *What of what has been lost can be recovered?*

In the domain of metaphysics, answers range from the centripetal visions of a Final Judgment (everything, at least for a moment and/or an eternity) to the liberating enslavement of Nietzsche's Eternal Recurrence (ditto—though not quite in the same way) across to the mothsmoke doctrine of *maya* (recover? what was *lost?* but my friend, it never was...). More pragmatic sallies at the same large problem include taxidermy, municipal archives, hard-hat archaeology, and modern historiography. Somewhere between those sweeping eschatological *strategies* (God, Time, the Void) and that clutch of mincing antiquarian-cum-academic *tactics* (lye soap, shovels, epigraphy) lie various mid-range programs for the creative constitution of nature, self, and society through acts of "recovery": e.g., environmentalism, psychoanalysis, nationalism. Each of these makes a recuperation of the effaced into a veritable gateway to our future.

Everything seems, eventually, to go away, to be broken, damaged, forgotten; to be devoured by time. Despite our needs and desires, very little can be restored. Thus the conditions of restoration are forever vexed: Who will do it? How? To what ends? On what authority? To what effects?

. . .

So the problem is large. Interestingly, however, much of it can be made to pass through a very small space. A tiny space. A space like the narrow strip of poplar panel to the immediate right of the Madonna in Duccio di Buoninsegna's *Maestà* of 1311. There, several hundred years of fluctuating temperature and humidity in the hilltop town of Siena (together with the other vicissitudes of existence—war, neglect, the equally destructive excesses of loving devotion) succeeded, by the early 1950s, in depriving the world of several square inches of paint that once represented a bit of patterned cloth folded over the throne of the Mother of Heaven.

What to do? What to do with this small hole—this *lacuna*, this blank, this discrete region of loss—pocking the world's artistic patrimony? *How to recover what was lost?*

The easy answer would seem to be: Paint it back

in. There's plenty of contextual evidence about how that strip once looked: it's a patterned cloth, after all. Patterns are, by definition, highly redundant. To put it in terms of information theory, they can still convey their message under very "noisy" conditions. Hence one can, without too much difficulty, reconstruct how the filigree of the cloth must have worked across the region in question. This would be an interpolation, to be sure, but one could feel relatively confident about the exercise.

And indeed, such minor restorative exercises—together with more fulsome interventions—have long been the work of that ill-defined community of practical custodians of the western artistic tradition. We call them "restorers" or "conservators" now, but for most of the history of painting in Europe they had no formal title or guild. They were artists and connoisseurs who, with varying degrees of success, took brush and palette to the work of their forebears for the purpose of touching up damaged goods. It was an empirical matter. A matter of *craft*. Of skill, to be sure, but also of knack. A sideline business, on the whole. Untheorized. Patrons might quibble about a tint or stroke. A sexton might complain about the cost. But this was not a formally polemical domain. Now and again, admittedly, an overzealous artist-restorer might get in trouble for carrying his gifts of pastiche all the way across to a culpable forgery, but this sort of showdown was uncommon. The navigable waters between fixing and faking were broad.

And it's here that the absence of a theory begins to intrude, since a proper distinction between "restoring" and "forging" is, when you stop and think about it, hard to articulate clearly. Are "restorations" simply small forgeries, contextually integrated, and done without (excessively) mercenary intent and/or malice? Such a back-of-the-envelope definition, however appealing, tends to trouble any tidy sense of the difference between recovery and invention, between history and fiction, and finally, perhaps, between truth and falsehood. Putting aside the important problem of how these matters were parsed by actors and thinkers across the historical periods in question (and ideas about the "original," the "copy," and the "fake" certainly changed a great deal between the Renaissance and the early twentieth century), one is left with what feels like, for better or worse, a philosophical problem. Maybe several.

Which brings us back to that little lacuna in Duccio's altarpiece, and to the philosophically inclined man who spent a good deal of time in the early 1950s looking at that hole, considering what was to be done: an Italian poet, critic, and aesthete named Cesare Brandi,

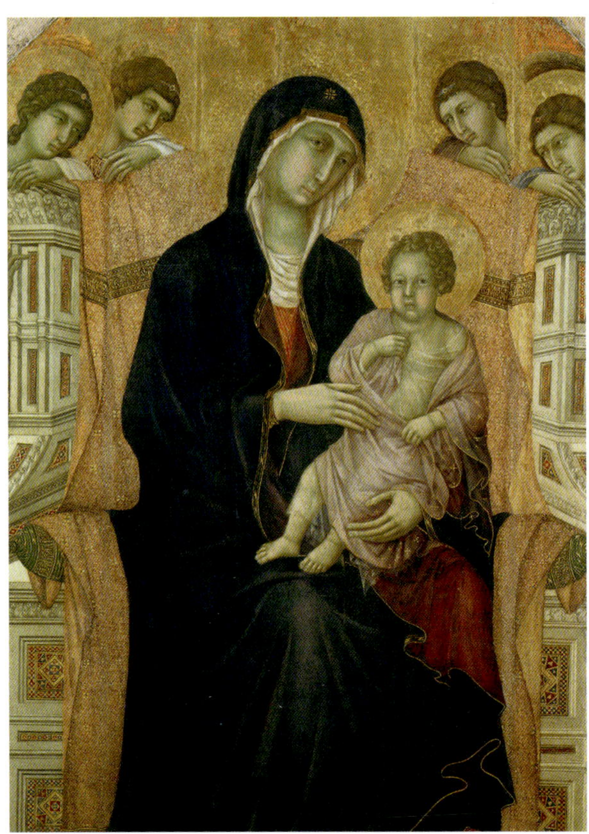

Shelving his early lyric poetry, he turned to writing in a sustained way on these durable topics, even as he acceded to positions of increasing prominence in the administrative structures of Italy's cultural establishment. Refined, brilliant, gay, a knotty thinker and yet a subtle institutional player in a complicated and dangerous political arena, Brandi was appointed in 1938 (at the tender age of thirty-two) as director of the newly created Istituto Centrale del Restauro in Rome. This well-endowed establishment, dedicated to the studious exaltation of Italy's artistic patrimony, had sprung fully grown from the forebrain of Mussolini's minister for culture, who, like his boss, churned with enthusiasm for a second renaissance of the greatness that was Italy. "Restoration" was emphatically a charged affair as the clouds darkened in the late 1930s.

When the smoke cleared in 1945, the importance of this project had increased dramatically, even if the situation had rather changed. Truculent classical visions of rebuilding Roman *imperium* and its Carrara-marble accoutrements (not necessarily Brandi's cup of tea, but certainly the preoccupation of those to whom he reported) had gone by the wayside. The shattered remains of countless monuments lay scattered about the piazzas of Italy's battered towns. Priceless frescos showed their war-wounds to the postwar world. Many of the greatest works of art of the cinquecento had to be brought up from the dank fruit cellars of Tuscan villas or exhumed from moldy catacombs. The need for *restoration* had perhaps never been as deeply felt as it was in Europe in those years.

It was in this context that Brandi—who, nimble through the chaos, had retained his post at the top of a phoenix-like post-Fascist Istituto—set to the task of building nothing less than a *theory of restoration*, a philosophically grounded analysis of the problem of artistic loss and recovery. And as he laid out his premises (the essential nature of a work of art, a coherent phenomenology of perception, an account of the ways that time inheres in a given art object), and elaborated his principles (of which more in a moment), he was uniquely positioned to operationalize his cogitations through the cultivation of *actual practices of art restoring*. Techniques. His philosophy in action. To be practiced by an institute that he controlled, which was then at work on an unprecedentedly vast project of artistic salvage—Brandi's formal brief. A very unusual situation. A philosopher with a mandate. And a staff.

who would become the most important theorist of *restauro*—restoration—in the twentieth century. He would become the brooding philosopher of *what could be recovered*.

Brandi was born in Siena in 1906, and he studied law before committing himself fully to the arts. By the early 1930s, after completing a thesis at the University of Florence on Italian Mannerism, he had curated a landmark exhibition of early Renaissance religious paintings. And shortly thereafter he won a distinguished appointment in the growing (Fascist) bureaucracy dedicated to the protection and promotion of Italy's vast heritage of classical masterworks. Like others of his generation in the Italian intelligentsia, this young belletrist and art historian found his way to the German idealists via the writings of the great aristocratic pessimist of Naples, Benedetto Croce, and in the mid-1930s Brandi began to fashion himself as a philosopher of aesthetics, laboring independently at the fundamental questions that dog literature, music, and the visual arts: What is the relationship between "form" and "content"? What is a "judgment of beauty"? What is the ultimate significance of artistic creation in human life?

---

above and opposite: Example of *tratteggio* in Duccio di Buoninsegna, *Majesty*, 1311 (detail). Courtesy Art Resource.

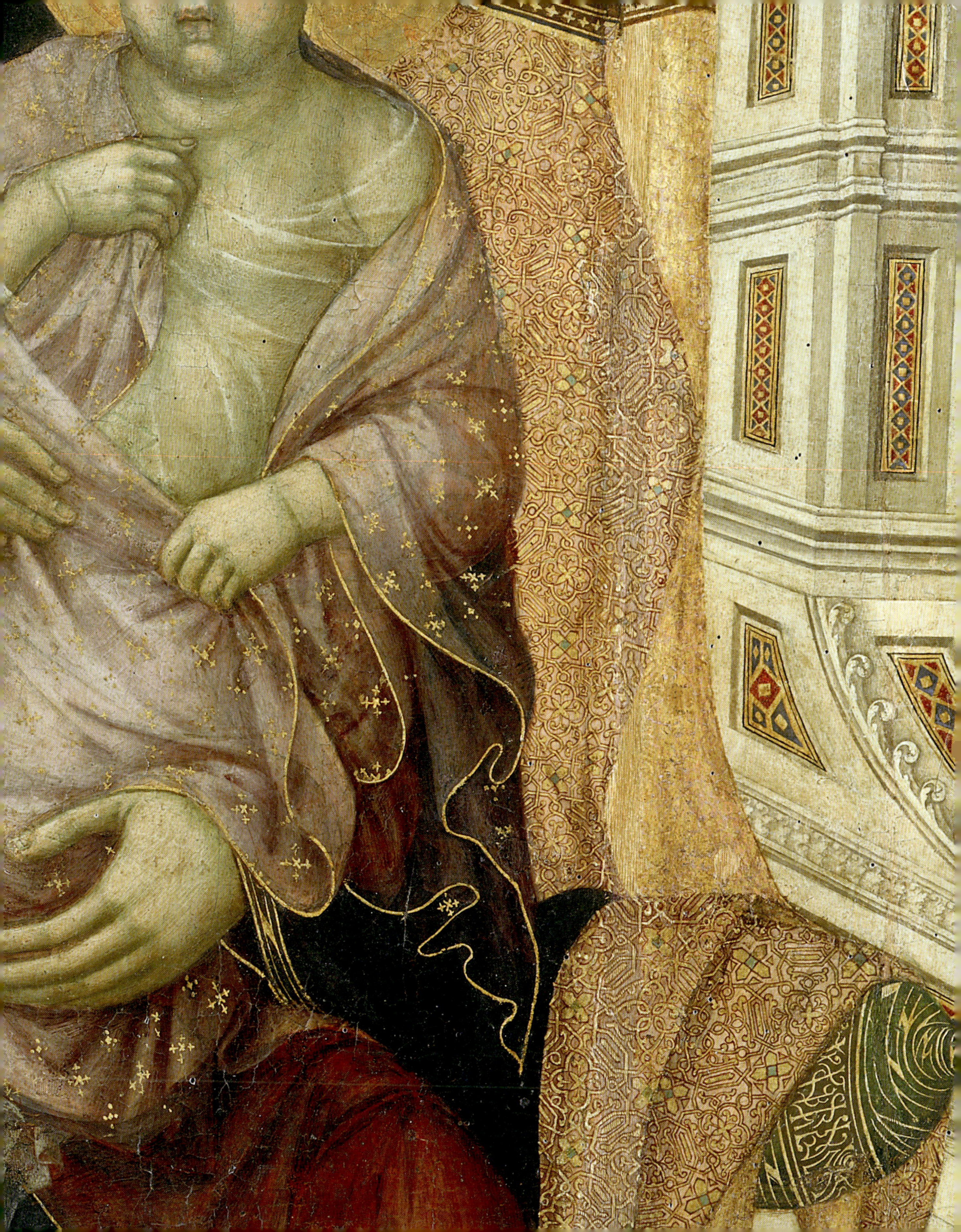

One can imagine catastrophe. The result was anything but. On the contrary, the result was beautiful, if also, in many ways, very strange.

. . .

The best way to approach Brandi's theory is probably via the painterly technique that embodied its central tenets and thereby realized its principles in pigment. This would be *tratteggio*, or, as it is sometimes called, *rigatino*. Both of these words mean something like "little line" in Italian, and in the context of art history they refer to the most important actual method developed at the Istituto Centrale del Restauro between 1947 and the mid-1950s. It is a method of "in-painting," a way of addressing lacunae in damaged panel paintings and frescos. It is a way of *recovering what was lost*.

For a sense of what *tratteggio* looks like, consider the detail reproduced here—the careful restoration of that unhappy blank strip in Duccio's long-suffering *Maestà*. What we get is very much a reconstruction of the patterned cloth. And yet, close observation reveals a peculiarly "ribbed" quality to the image across the restored region, a distinctive patterning of the new brushstrokes which are thereby set off from the original. This is *tratteggio* in all its glory. The technique stipulates a set of highly artificial constraints on the brushwork of the restorer, who is required to make exclusively parallel, rectilinear hachures of fixed length by means of an exceedingly fine brush. Each stroke must consist of a single charging of the brush—ideally with a "pure" hue (the most rigorous applications of the method actually demand the exclusive use of a fixed range of fundamental, unmixed colors)—and a single gesture of the hand. Color blending on the canvas or panel is strictly prohibited, as, indeed, is any overlapping of strokes whatsoever. In its purest formulation, all *tratteggio* in-painting must be built up on a white gesso ground using only the optical effects of perceptual color-mixing dear to pointillists like Seurat or Signac— or, to place the approach more firmly in its 1950s context, dear to the developers of the color televisions then coming to market for the first time.

The technique—codified as an actual practice by a pair of gifted artist-restorers at the Istituto, Paolo and Laura Mora, who worked under Brandi's supervision (he was not a painter)—amounts to a fascinating mash-up of high-modernist occularity and premodern mimesis. All in the name of *recovery*.

. . .

Okay. Restoration by means of something like *pixilation*.

Interesting. But, um, why?

The answer goes to the heart of Brandi's conceptualization of art itself—to the heart of his efforts to integrate commitments to historical truth, scientific precision, and aesthetic experience. In essence, Brandi believed that an act of *restauro* could go wrong in two fundamental ways. On the one hand, an "empirical" restorer could pick up his brush and paint in the missing bits—using his soul, his eye, and his gift. This was, in Brandi's view, nothing more or less than defacement—effectively graffiti. The "better" such work was (the more invisible) the worse it became, since it imperceptibly corrupted the original and defiled, perhaps irreversibly, the plastic instantiation of the veritable *work*—the thing itself, its quasi-sacred sensual reality. All merely empirical restoration was thus indeed *forgery* plain and simple: falsehood, the unholy enemy of art and life.

On the other hand, there were the "archaeological" restorers—positivists, men of science. These types tended to be scrupulous, and ascetically devoted to the unembellished reconstruction of what could be reconstructed. If they were working on an ancient statue, they reassembled the shards they could find, and that was it. If they were working on a damaged painting, they might stitch up a torn canvas, or stabilize the lacunae with wax or plaster, but that was it. "Reconstruct" the missing bits of the image? Never. These museological undertakers were too committed to the scientistic ideal of the "bare fact" to grasp the (higher) aesthetic ideals at play. Which is to say, they failed to understand that restoring a work of art is fundamentally different from restoring the puzzle bits of a broken millstone.

Enter the philosopher of aesthetics. A work of art possesses, according to Brandi, a dual nature: on the one hand, its existential reality (its thingness); and on the other, its pure reality (its bid to transcend that thingness). It is its measure of the latter, of course, that actually makes a given object a work of art. *What art is* (cue soundtrack of German idealism) is the mysterious/paradoxical/magnificent *presence of transcendence in mere things*. Made, but freed from their mere becoming by their reach for eternity, such objects exist in time (as objects) but also defy (as works of art) simply being pinned to the past on a timeline, since they possess a transhistorical power to present to a consciousness, in any given present, *reality as such*: call it "Consciousness" (or Spirit, or *Geist*, or whatever).

This sort of aesthetic theorizing trepidates on the threshold of the ineffable. Analytic philosophers tend to dismiss it all as so much breathless verbiage. Even a sympathetic reader must concede that the technicalities get to be a genuine headache in a hurry. There's some Hegel in Brandi's account, for sure. But maybe, in the end, even more Kant. People argue about influences and inclinations. And Brandi's own thinking on these questions evolved: by the 1960s, he was talking about Husserl, Heidegger, even Derrida. You'd have to be a card-carrying Continental philosopher to sort it all out, and even those folks aren't sure it wholly hangs together. But the basic point is this: artworks, if they are anything, are special kinds of historico-material objects, and this specialness resides, somehow, in their own ambition to transcend their mere historicity and their mere materiality. This sort of idealism is not an absurd position, however mystical it may finally be. Indeed, one might argue that the burden lies on those who have an interest in art but find all this unpersuasive to tell us why they care about paintings, sculpture, and the like. Why not everything else?

But put the merits of Brandi's core theory of aesthetics aside. His propositions granted, the "restoration" of artworks becomes a very particular business. *Such an exercise must be formally faithful to their double nature as material and aesthetic objects*. Which is to say, any restoration becomes, for Brandi, the *materialization of a critical interpretation*. The empirical restorers of old, the over-painting hacks, failed to understand the essential self-reflective program of *critique* (the investigation of the conditions of possibility of the work of art as such, and thus of anything like its "restoration"), and the archaeologists, steeped in a crude historical positivism, failed to grasp the demands of *interpretation*—failed to see that merely assembling the fragments was to fail to reassemble the work, which required the loving and sensitive reconstitution (to the degree possible) of its essential unity as a work of art, the reconstitution of its *aesthetic reality*. Any "scientific" restoration that left the viewer distractingly aware of the material nature of the object *qua object* (lacunae, visible modern structural elements supporting the ancient fragments, etc.) actually risked stripping the work of its aesthetic power altogether, in effect demoting it from the sphere of art to the world of mere things. Any "artistic" restoration that tried to cover up its tracks (through invisible integration and/or pastiche) made a mockery of the essential nature of art by violating the work's existential reality and absolute specificity— concepts without which art itself was, in Brandi's view, unintelligible.

So what about *tratteggio*? *Tratteggio* embodied exactly these principles of "critical/interpretive"

restoration. The aim was to *reconstitute the aesthetic unity of the work* (to give the viewer the integral and total experience of the work with full force) while *scrupulously honoring the work's material reality*. From a distance, we see a complete image of the Madonna on her well-draped and sumptuous throne—we experience Duccio's "work of art." Then, coming up close, we discern without difficulty the interpretive interpolation of the lacuna that has assisted in affording us this complete aesthetic encounter—we reckon with the material, historical object: Duccio's *work*. At a distance: *integrity* in the holistic sense (since we see the image as a whole). Up close: *integrity* in the ethical sense (since at that range the marks resolve themselves as an interpretive intervention, and we can attend without risk of confusion on Duccio's veritable *oeuvre* in its historical specificity, discern the scarring of time upon his labor, see *what he did*, and, crucially, *what he did not do*). When we are back at suitable distance, those little parallel marks again body forth the *unità potenziale* of the masterpiece—its "potential unity," the mystical integrity that inheres in a true work of art, and in any recoverable component thereof.

· · ·

That was the idea, anyway. And it was an idea, and a practice, that held sway in Italy for much of the postwar period (Brandi lived until 1988, and remained a sovereign force in the peninsula's artistic life to the end). *Tratteggio* even spawned schismatic sects and foreign emulators. In the 1960s, the Florentines, under the leadership of Umberto Baldini, cultivated a rival practice they called "chromatic abstraction," which, thrown contemptuously into the teeth of Brandi's (Roman) school at the time, nevertheless looks in retrospect like a very modest departure. It permitted the particulate hachures to cross; it admitted of some shifts in orientation of the resulting grid; it allowed a wee bit more coloristic latitude. Later, French and Belgian traditions arose that deployed the same general approach (what came to be known as "visible" in-painting, the general term for all the techniques that relied on ocular integration), but used pointillist dots or freer *macchie*, the technical term for a brushwork of specks and splotches.

On the whole, though, all of these approaches have now mostly passed from grace. There are still a few practitioners of the art of *tratteggio*, but only a small number of curators would currently consider submitting a work of significance to this treatment, and several famous examples of visible in-painting are these days widely regarded with horror (signally Cimabue's

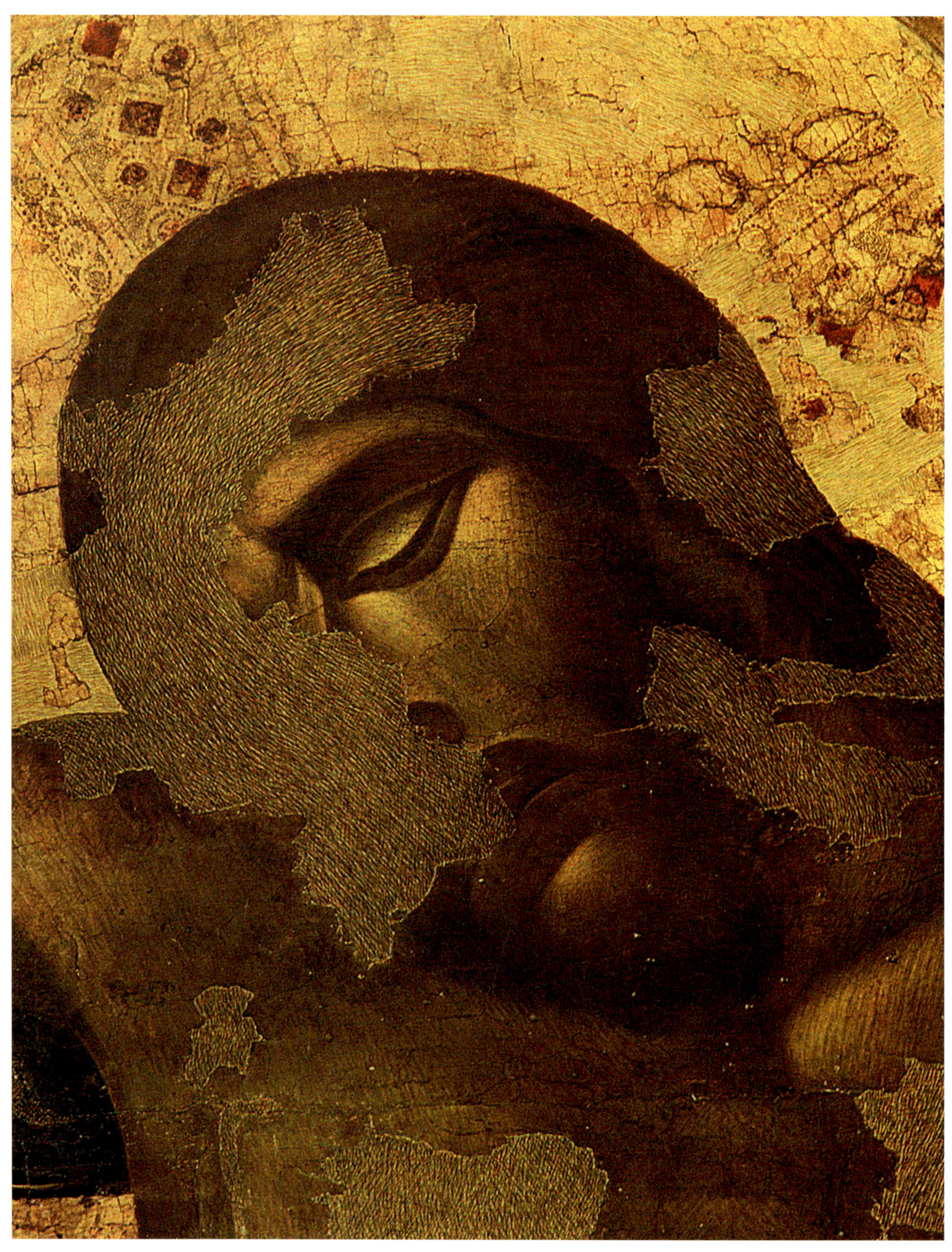

Detail of Cimabue's *Crucifix* (1287–1288) after restoration, showing the use of chromatic abstraction (*astrazione cromatica*).

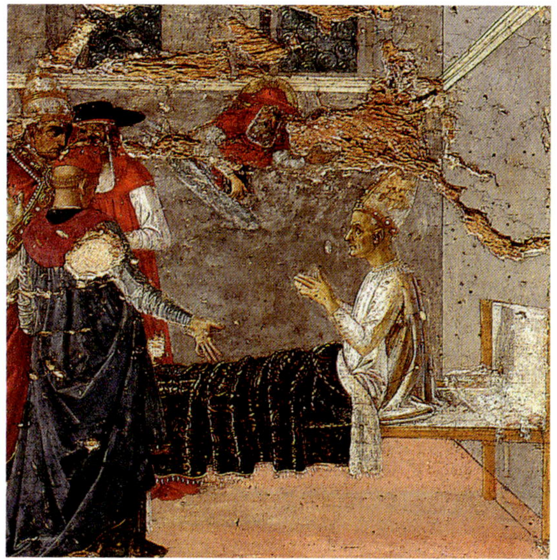 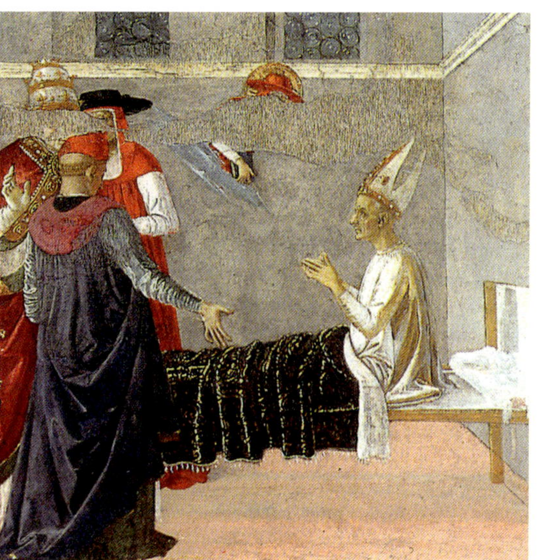

Pietro Perugino's *Scenes from the Life of St Jerome* (1495), during cleaning and after restoration. Nineteenth-century "empirical" in-paintings were removed and replaced with a combination of modulated *tratteggio* (with more varied colors) for architectural elements and neutral gray *tratteggio* for figures and faces.

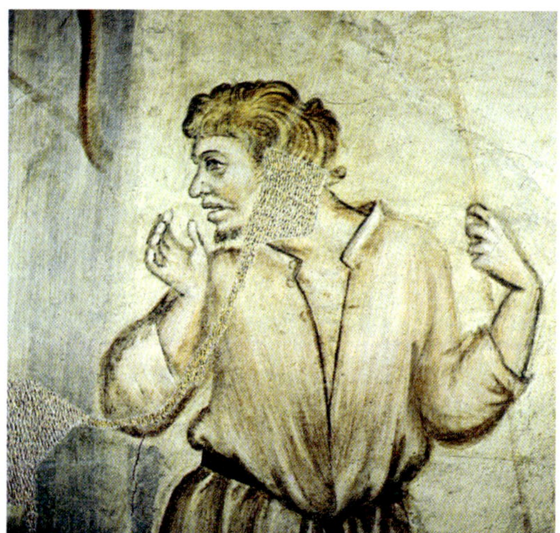

Example of the use of chromatic abstraction to fill a lacuna in an early fourteenth-century fresco in the Velluti Chapel of the Basilica of Santa Croce, Florence.

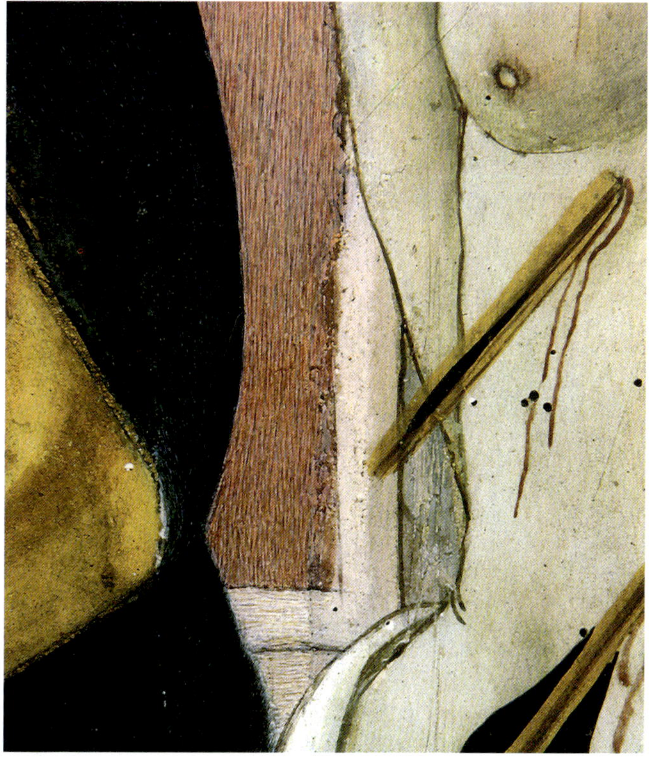

Detail of the restored *Enthroned Madonna* (fifteenth century), attributed to the Master of San Miniato, in the Pieve di San Bartolomeo at Pomino near Florence. The in-painting shown here (chromatic abstraction) reflects four distinct passes with four separate hues: the first yellow, the second orange-red, the third blue, and the last in tiny quantities of black to darken the overall effect.

Crocifisso, badly damaged in the Florence floods of 1966, and restored with extensive chromatic abstraction). Today, even in Italy, lacunae are, again, routinely handled by means of *invisible* in-painting, the kind of restoration that hides its tracks—exactly what Brandi loudly denounced.

Interestingly, though, even the new "empirical" in-painters mostly consider themselves heirs to the great Cesare Brandi, and he is still invoked as the founder of the theory of art restoration. His legacy in the field is now understood to lie less in *tratteggio* per se (which, after all, he did not really invent—that honor properly belongs to his staff), and more in his concern with reversibility (*tratteggio* was uniquely undertaken in watercolor), and his ideas about the multiple temporalities of a work of art. Extending his central analysis of an artwork's dual nature, he argued that the restorer had an obligation to honor both the historical moment of the work's making and the historical time that it had gathered—that passage of time marked in the object itself and inextricable from its presence to consciousness. Brandi used the distinction to argue against excessively invasive efforts to restore works to their "original condition," since their patina had become part of our experience of the works themselves. The philosopher of recovery had, it turned out, a very refined feel for decay.

In fact, as concerned as he was with *restoration*, Brandi's life was, in effect, a long and complicated love affair with loss. As he got older, he would come to advocate that every *restauro* should preserve a small region of the original untouched, so that over time, through repeated restorations, a work would gradually become an intricate archive of its own ruin—an emerging fugue of temporalities, here hesitating, here in recapitulation, here performing counterpoint to its own eternal cadence. *Voilà*: the play of loss and recovery as the *work of art itself*.

And this, finally, may be the right way to think of *tratteggio*. It looks like a tactic for recovery, but it may well be a strategy for loss. Or maybe it's something *in-between*, a way of filling in that space between repair and resignation, method and metaphysics. How it works may depend, in the end, on *where you stand*: how near, how far. It is all this, I think, that gives me a shiver, looking at these works. In those small spaces one can—stepping close, stepping back—sense a roiling ambition to reconceive not just the past, but how we access it, and why: what we owe the dead, and ourselves, when we try to picture what is lost. Thought of this way, as a metaphor for historical practice per

se, *tratteggio* creatively destabilizes conventional distinctions between historical fiction and the footnoted monograph, and inflects the act of recovering the past with spiritual (and aesthetic) significance. What would it be to write history using a version of this technique? To "fill in" what is missing by means of the textual equivalent of this peculiar convention? Suddenly it seems there is a great deal of work to be done.

So much for *tratteggio* as visual historiography. What about *tratteggio* as visual art? Here I would argue that these restorations merit reconsideration as significant twentieth-century artworks. Call the school "epistemic expressionism"—a visual idiom imbued with the torments of beauty in an age of truth. Indeed, one might go so far as to claim that visible in-painting has given us the only significant high allegorical paintings of modernism. How else to understand these hybrid creations if not as tiny, elaborate *masques* of the central problem of the modernist program: that uneasy, recursive dialectic between tradition and innovation, freedom and history. "Revolution," of course, means a *turn that brings you back to your original position*. The avant-garde is forever at work forgetting this. And remembering.

. . .

What of what has been lost can be recovered? Looking at that little strip of the *Maestà*—up close, and then from a distance—one wants to say: "*You can, you must, recover ... the loss.*"

> *What kind of taste and organs must those people have, who really prefer the adulterate enjoyments of the town to the genuine pleasures of a country retreat?*
> —Tobias Smollett, *The Expedition of Humphry Clinker*, 1771

Around 1750 on the outskirts of Paris, designers at King Louis XV's porcelain manufactory began producing a type of cup for drinking milk known as the "milk goblet," or *gobelet à lait*. Available in two sizes, the cups had one or two handles and a cover to keep the milk warm. They were often decorated with country scenes and painted in pastel hues like "Pompadour pink," named after Louis XV's mistress Madame de Pompadour, who was one of the factory's most important patrons. In the 1750s, milk goblets became popular among the French nobility and the court, and they were also given away as gifts to foreign dignitaries.[1]

Part of the cup's appeal stemmed from the material out of which it was made. Beginning in the fifteenth century, porcelain from China had been imported into Europe in ever-growing quantities, and it was fiercely coveted among European elites, so much so that in 1717 the ruler of Saxony, Augustus the Strong, traded six hundred of his cavalrymen to the king of Prussia in exchange for 151 porcelain Ming vases. The soldiers became known as the Porcelain Regiment.[2] For centuries, European artisans had struggled to imitate this Asian "white gold," but it wasn't until 1709 that the Saxon alchemist Johann Friedrich Böttger figured out how to manufacture true or hard-paste porcelain, which was done by combining a hard, feldspathic rock known as petuntse with kaolin, a white clay common to both Asia and Europe.

Böttger was put in charge of Augustus the Strong's new factory at Meissen, the first European producer of hard-paste porcelain. Meissen's success spurred other European rulers to found their own factories and attempt to divine or steal the formula. Louis XV's manufactory had been founded in 1740 at Vincennes near Paris, and in 1756 it was moved to Sèvres on the opposite side of the city. Although the Sèvres factory didn't begin producing true porcelain until the late 1760s— shortly after French manufacturers stumbled upon a large deposit of kaolin near Limoges—in the early years they developed an artificial soft-paste version made of clay and powdered glass that was admired by wealthy

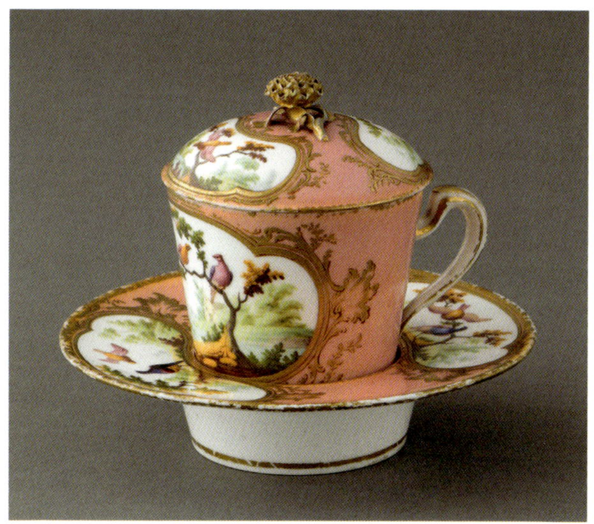

Sèvres milk goblet (*Gobelet à lait*) with recessed saucer, sometimes also known as a *trembleuse*, ca. 1759. Photo Réunion des musées nationaux / Art Resource.

collectors across Europe. The milk goblet shown above was made using this soft-paste technique, adding to its status as an object of desire and prestige.

However, it was the milk cup's function that truly ensured its popularity among French high society in the 1750s. While drinking fresh milk is ubiquitous in the West today, it was a novelty, at least among adults, in early modern Europe, when people of all classes were more likely to consume dairy products in the form of butter or cheese. Prior to the nineteenth-century development of pasteurization and refrigeration, fresh milk spoiled too quickly to be regularly or widely consumed, especially among city residents. Milk was, however, prescribed as a medicinal remedy in antiquity and the Renaissance, and this practice was revived in eighteenth-century Europe as part of a back-to-nature health craze aimed at urban elites, and elite women in particular.[3]

The milk cure was associated with the neo-Hippocratic revival of medicine, which, according to historian William Coleman, had become by 1750 "an integral part of a new and largely secular moral order."[4] Supplanting earlier medical theories that focused solely on the body's internal dynamics, the new Hippocratic code emphasized diet, hygiene, environment, and lifestyle. Eighteenth-century physicians who subscribed to this code—among them Samuel Tissot, who corresponded with Jean-Jacques Rousseau and wrote bestselling treatises on the perils of masturbation, high-class urban living, and excessive scholarly activity—urged their predominantly elite patients to repair to the countryside and rid themselves of the city's deleterious influences by taking in fresh air and sunlight, enjoying moderate exercise, and consuming milk and other wholesome foods. Tissot believed that this regimen would salvage the morals as well as the health of his patients by bringing them closer to a prelapsarian state of nature. It would also put them in contact with the rural peasantry, whose rustic diet and idealized devotion to work and family Tissot, in a utopian fashion, encouraged his followers to emulate.[5]

Milk, a substance that Rousseau identified with pastoral purity and the "natural" innocence and sweetness of women, was an essential part of the back-to-nature health campaign.[6] Although physicians debated its efficacy in treating certain illnesses and constitutions, milk was generally believed to function as a non-violent purgative that penetrated and opened the body's channels, allowing fresh air to enter and toxins to exit. It could also be used to remove obstructions in the lungs, chest, and bowels, returning the body to its optimal balance or flow. In an article on milk for the *Encyclopédie* (1751–1765), the French royal physician Gabriel-François Venel touted its success in treating nerve disorders along with chest and stomach ailments, fever, gout, and venereal disease. Venel preferred to prescribe cow's milk, while other physicians maintained that ass's, goat's, or even human breast milk was superior. He also recommended that fragile patients drink whey, or the watery part of milk that remains after curdling, because it was easier to digest than whole milk. Whey was considered especially good for those suffering from the "hypochondriacal and hysterical illnesses" that were thought to be alarmingly on the rise in this period, notably among women.[7]

The *Encyclopédie*'s advice, echoed in publications from the 1750s to the 1780s, stimulated a mania for the milk diet among aristocrats and Enlightenment *philosophes* alike. Diderot and Voltaire both tried it, and Rousseau enjoyed bathing in whey and also drinking it. By the mid-1780s, the Parisian journalist Louis-Sébastien Mercier could comment ruefully on how "the rich eat much less than they used to ... you may see your host, at the head of his magnificent table, dismally sipping a glass of milk," and he could also report on strenuous efforts to import in-demand Swiss dairy cows to Paris, which city residents believed would give them "a new lease on life" until they were disappointed to discover that the Alpine creatures could not thrive "on our thin French fields."[8] Undaunted by such challenges, Parisian physicians and businessmen parlayed the siren call of nature into lucrative enterprises, churning out

testimonials, treating scores of gullible patients, and designing alluring products like rouge made from vegetable dye and the *tronchine*, a short, unstructured dress that women could wear while walking outdoors. (The *tronchine* was developed by Théodore Tronchin, who treated Voltaire and the French royal family.) For those who could not obtain fresh milk—or who had no wish to leave the city—substitute remedies were devised such as "Franchipane," a milk-and-herb extract invented by the German physician Friedrich Hoffmann that promised nature in a bottle.[9]

At the high end of this market, the porcelain milk goblet offered the possibility of returning to nature in an artful manner, while also participating in the latest health trends. The Sèvres cup shown on the previous page embodies a rose-colored vision of country life, and was engineered expressly with the milk cure in mind. First, it was large enough to contain the pint (*chopine*) of milk that patients were advised to consume once or twice daily. The handle aided an infirm drinker's shaky grasp, and it also kept hands free of the cup's hot surface, since milk was often served warm to promote relaxation and digestion. The cover conserved this warmth and kept the liquid free of wig powder or other contaminants that could fall in during the morning ritual of the *toilette*, when milk was frequently served.

The most striking visual element of this particular milk goblet may be its recessed or "socketed" saucer, which allows the cup to fit snugly into its base. Introduced by the Sèvres factory in 1759, this type of saucer was apparently designed to prevent anxious or feverish milk drinkers—especially elite women suffering from nervous disorders like hysteria or "the vapors"—from knocking the cup over and shattering it. The cup-and-saucer ensemble is sometimes referred to as a "*trembleuse*," an eighteenth-century term that evoked the trembling hands of the fragile patients who gripped these vessels.[10] The seeming urgency for such a cup is evident in the many eighteenth-century novels that feature overly sensitive characters, usually women, who are so overcome by emotional travails or the pressures of urban life that they have been reduced to a perpetual state of nervous trembling. Two of the best-known examples are Samuel Richardson's heroines Pamela and Clarissa, whose eponymous novels were published in 1740 and 1747–48, respectively. Clarissa admits at one point to being so "choked with vapours" that she cannot finish a milk-and-tea concoction she is given for her health, while Pamela describes her hands shaking so badly that she spills a cup of hot chocolate during an episode in which she agonizes over marrying her

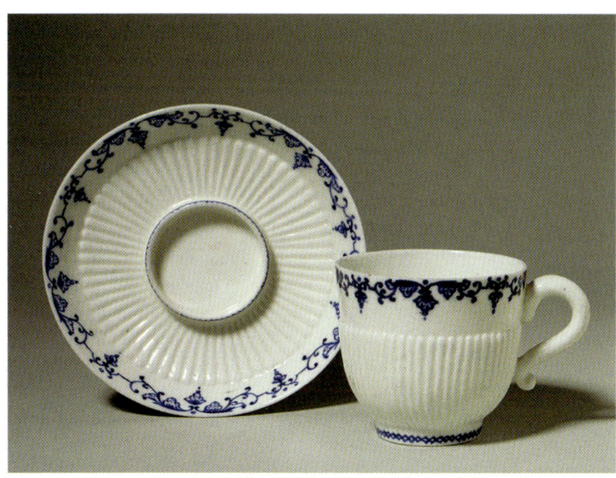

Trembleuse cup and saucer from the Saint-Cloud porcelain factory, ca. 1730–1750. Courtesy Victoria and Albert Museum, London.

wealthy but possibly unscrupulous employer, Mr. B.[11]

An earlier type of *trembleuse* cup had been invented in the late seventeenth century at Saint-Cloud, France's first commercially viable producer of soft-paste porcelain. The Saint-Cloud *trembleuse* was designed for consuming coffee, tea, and chocolate: exotic beverages that had only recently been made available in France and were initially thought to possess restorative or medicinal properties. A treatise published on these beverages in 1685 attested to their ability to alleviate gout, the vapors, infertility, and consumption.[12] Unlike the Sèvres cup's recessed saucer, the Saint-Cloud saucer had a raised central ring or "gallery" for securing the cup that resembled a *mancerina*, a cup-and-saucer combination used primarily for drinking chocolate. The *mancerina* was named after the Marqués de Mancera, the Spanish viceroy of Peru from 1639 to 1648, who had helped import chocolate from the New World and drank large quantities of it himself to treat his palsy.[13]

Most Saint-Cloud *trembleuses* are ornamented with blue and white arabesque motifs that were fashionable in France in the late seventeenth century. The shape and color of these cups derived from Chinese porcelain prototypes and called to mind the exotic nature of the beverages they contained. As *trembleuses* grew in popularity in the early eighteenth century, newly minted porcelain manufactories scrambled to create their own versions of these vessels. The most elaborate were the *trembleuses* made by the Du Paquier factory in Vienna (founded in 1718), which featured an intricate, pierced gallery that showcased the fragile nature of both the material and the consumer.[14] Clients purchased *trembleuse* cups not just

because of their usefulness but also because they had the ability to suggest an owner's delicate constitution or nervous sensitivity, which became what historian Roy Porter has described as a "badge of gentility" among the eighteenth-century European elite.[15]

In the first half of the eighteenth century, coffee, tea, and chocolate became all the rage in Europe. Some members of the Enlightenment medical community, however, began denouncing these substances, arguing that they could actually provoke some of the ailments they were formerly believed to alleviate.[16] Coffee, tea, and chocolate were also tied to the urbane lifestyle that mid-century physicians and social reformers began widely to condemn as physically and morally enervating. Though these drinks remained popular, they were eclipsed after 1750 by new beverages that extolled the regenerative virtues of country living, including milk served by itself rather than combined with these products.

One of the most fervent devotees of the back-to-nature trend in France was Madame de Pompadour, Louis XV's mistress from 1745 until her death in 1764. Pompadour suffered from poor health throughout her years at court—her chronic fevers, nervous attacks, and lung problems are amply documented in court memoirs—and she spent much of her time in the company of her physician, François Quesnay, who encouraged her to drink milk and adopt the new natural remedies. (Pompadour and Quesnay co-hosted a salon at Versailles attended by such cutting-edge intellectuals as Diderot and d'Alembert, where the new medical theories were discussed.)[17] A 1758 portrait of Pompadour by her favorite artist, François Boucher, depicts her promoting the rejuvenating effects of nature while

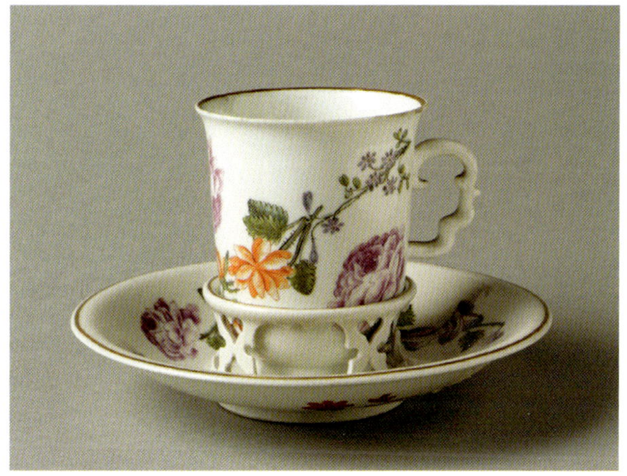

Trembleuse cup and saucer from the Du Paquier porcelain factory, ca. 1730–1735. Courtesy Victoria and Albert Museum, London.

she reads a book, possibly one of the many medical treatises in her library. One of these treatises, Antonio Cocchi's *The Pythagorean Diet, of Vegetables Only, Conducive to the Preservation of Health and the Cure of Diseases* (1743), endorsed the healing power of nature, vegetables, and milk.

Pompadour acquired several milk goblets in the 1750s, and between 1759 and her death in 1764 she seems to have purchased every *trembleuse* cup with a recessed saucer that the Sèvres factory produced.[18] She took her therapeutic regimen to even more lavish extremes by commissioning quasi-rural retreats near the royal palaces of Versailles, Fontaine-bleau, and Compiègne, where she could escape to pastoral seclusion for an afternoon or more. These retreats, known as "hermitages," were named after rural huts inhabited by recluses or monks seeking isolation and spiritual contemplation. Pompadour's refuges, by contrast, proclaimed a new religion of nature and were dedicated to purifying the body as well as the mind. Along with sizeable gardens, they all featured cow stables and dairies for the production of milk and whey, which she consumed on a regular basis.

Visited by courtiers throughout the 1750s, Pompadour's dairies, like her hermitages, represented an elegant and sophisticated vision of rural life. They were airy pavilions outfitted with marble tables, statues of milkmaids, and porcelain milk goblets that she purchased from her Parisian art dealer Lazare Duvaux. As spaces in which to "perform," as much as participate, in the new cultural trends, they belonged to a type of garden building known as the pleasure dairy, or *laiterie d'agrément*, that became popular among the French aristocracy around the mid-eighteenth century. Following Pompadour's example, royal women like Marie-Antoinette and Josephine de Beauharnais built pleasure dairies to flaunt their superior health, taste, and commitment to the land, modeling themselves on Rousseau's virtuous heroine Julie, who runs her own pastoral community and dairy at Clarens in the bestselling novel *Julie, ou La nouvelle Héloïse* (1761).

Marie-Antoinette's pleasure dairy, built in the 1780s as part of her faux-rustic hamlet (*Hameau*) at Versailles, exemplified this building type in its blend of outward simplicity and interior refinement—representing an architectural analogue of the pastoral literary mode. Often dismissed as the wasteful folly of a frivolous queen, the *Hameau*'s dairy was in fact part of a larger trend of similar structures created during this time on the grounds of palaces, country estates, and even in the gardens of wealthy Parisians, and

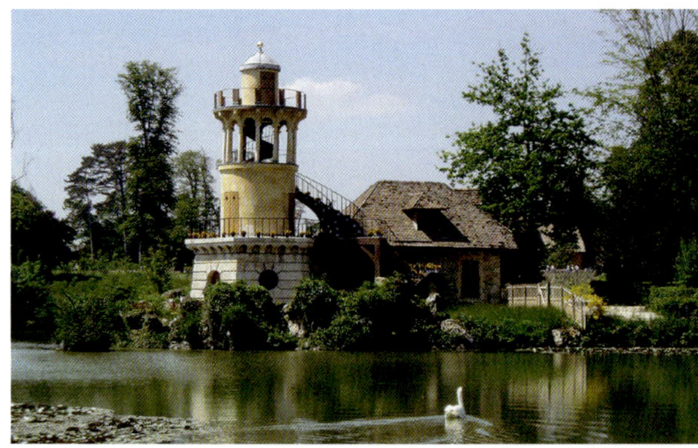

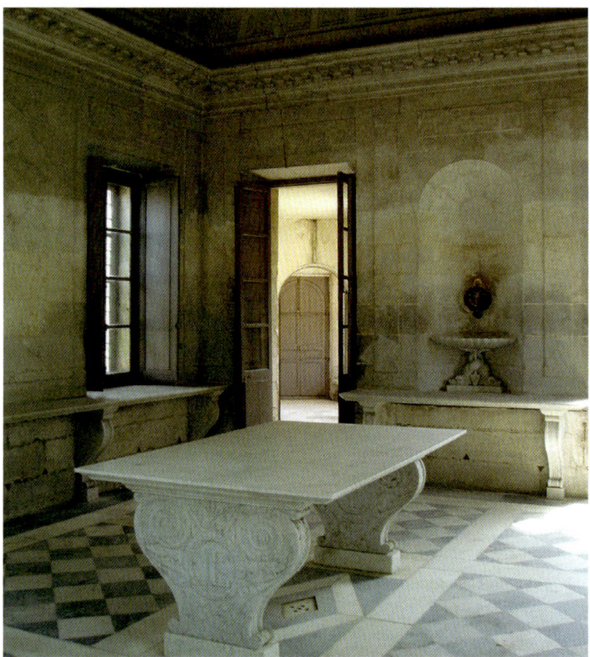

Exterior and interior of Marie-Antoinette's pleasure dairy, Hameau de Versailles, designed by Richard Mique, ca. 1783–1787. Photos Meredith Martin.

they remain important in our understanding of the creative relationship between the aristocracy and leading artists and architects of the day, including Hubert Robert, François Boucher, and Claude-Nicolas Ledoux. Moreover, pleasure dairies allowed elite owners to experience the pleasures, and embrace the values, of rural life without having to abandon their urban-oriented lifestyles or their courtly responsibilities.

These buildings and their stylish gardens drew harsh complaint, however, from Enlightenment reformers and physicians, who worried that their owners were mocking the rhetoric of pastoral retreat or turning it into a bankrupt performance. In the 1770s Louis de Carmontelle capitalized on this anxiety by writing a satirical play about a Parisian noblewoman who fakes a hysterical attack so that her doctor will prescribe a milk diet, conning her husband into whisking her away to their country house just so she can entertain her friends there.[19] Marie-Antoinette's critics went much further by accusing her of using her garden retreat, with its connotations of feminine virtue, as a haven for indulging in degenerate sex acts with her male relatives and female friends. Rumors about the queen's misconduct in her gardens appeared in pornographic pamphlets written about her before the Revolution, and they reappeared during her trial of 1793, shortly before she was guillotined.[20] Attacks against Marie-Antoinette may have been in the extreme, but in the late eighteenth century it was common to label a woman unnatural or corrupt if she did not embrace the "genuine pleasures" of country living and the attendant values of domesticity, or, worse yet, if she was thought to fake a sincere attachment to those values for her own selfish ends.

Medical treatises published in this period, many of which were written by physicians attached to the court, encouraged husbands and colleagues to forcibly transplant women to the countryside if they refused to go gently in order to be "cured." One of these treatises, D. T. de Bienville's *Nymphomania or Treatise on the Uterine Furies* (1771)—"uterine furies" being a popular term for the sexually specific form of hysteria or the vapors—reads more like a gothic novel than a scientific tract. It is filled with scurrilous accounts of wayward women whom the author had personally saved by insisting on a strict regimen of country isolation, warm baths, and milk. In one such account involving an oversexed teenager named "Eléonore," Dr. Bienville describes how he delivered this "monstrous," perpetually "trembling" young girl to his own country house and fed her a purifying diet of white meat and milk while also administering daily injections of milk into her vagina, which to his satisfaction made her clitoris recede.[21] By the end of his tale, he proudly proclaims that Eléonore is not only completely cured but that she has also re-entered society and found a husband. Bienville's treatise underscores the extent to which the back-to-nature campaign could be used as a tool by men to police women, to delimit their identity and their desire, and to define their "natural" place in society—anticipating the treatment of so-called hysterical women in the nineteenth century and beyond.

Anti-royal pamphlets also accused Marie-Antoinette of suffering from "uterine furies."[22] In an effort to reform the queen's image and extricate her from her sullied gardens and *Hameau*, Louis XVI's building director, Charles-Claude Flahaut de la Billarderie, Comte

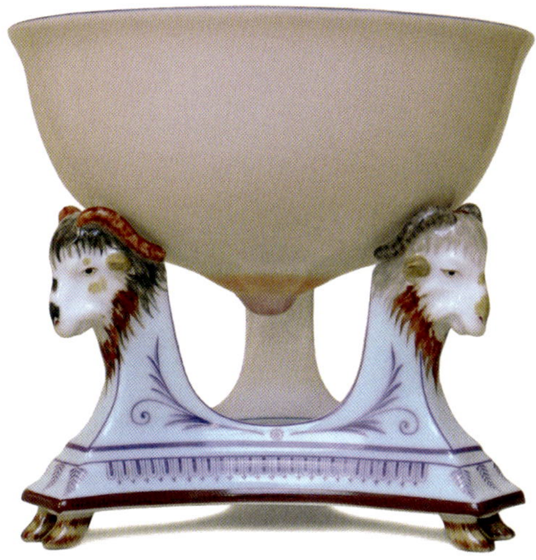

Replica of the Sèvres "breast cup" (*jatte téton*) designed by Jean-Jacques Lagrenée for the Queen's Dairy at Rambouillet, 1786–1787. Photo Claire Lehmann.

d'Angiviller, commissioned a second dairy around 1785 for Marie-Antoinette at the royal estate of Rambouillet, where the king spent his days hunting. The Rambouillet dairy, whose exterior resembled a neoclassical temple, was intended to convey social, political, and aesthetic renewal on a grand scale. Inside was a womblike grotto crowned by a statue of the mythological nymph Amalthea, who according to Ovid's *Fasti* had nursed the infant Jupiter with goat's milk while he was separated from his mother. Surrounding her were plaques, made of a milky marble, depicting similarly dutiful women performing domestic tasks like churning butter, shearing sheep, and breastfeeding children—referring to a contemporary campaign of social renewal, promoted by Rousseau among others, that entreated Frenchwomen to nurse their own children instead of hiring wet nurses.

Breastfeeding and (animal) milk consumption were further aligned in a suite of antique-inspired Sèvres porcelain that d'Angiviller commissioned for the dairy, which included a milk goblet shaped like a woman's breast. To drink from it, one had to lift the flesh-colored cup carefully from its tripod base, cradle the breast in both hands, and sip milk from the rim. In its design and use, the Rambouillet breast cup embodied both the yearning for regeneration and the erotic impulses associated with the milk cure that reformers were

---

overleaf: Louis de Carmontelle, *The Farm Girls* (Madame de la Houze and Mademoiselle de Longueil), ca. 1782. Photo Réunion des Musées Nationaux / Art Resource. In this gouache, Carmontelle depicts two high-society Parisian women drinking milk and getting back to nature in an artful fashion, a practice that he lampooned in his play *La Rosière* (written in the 1770s).

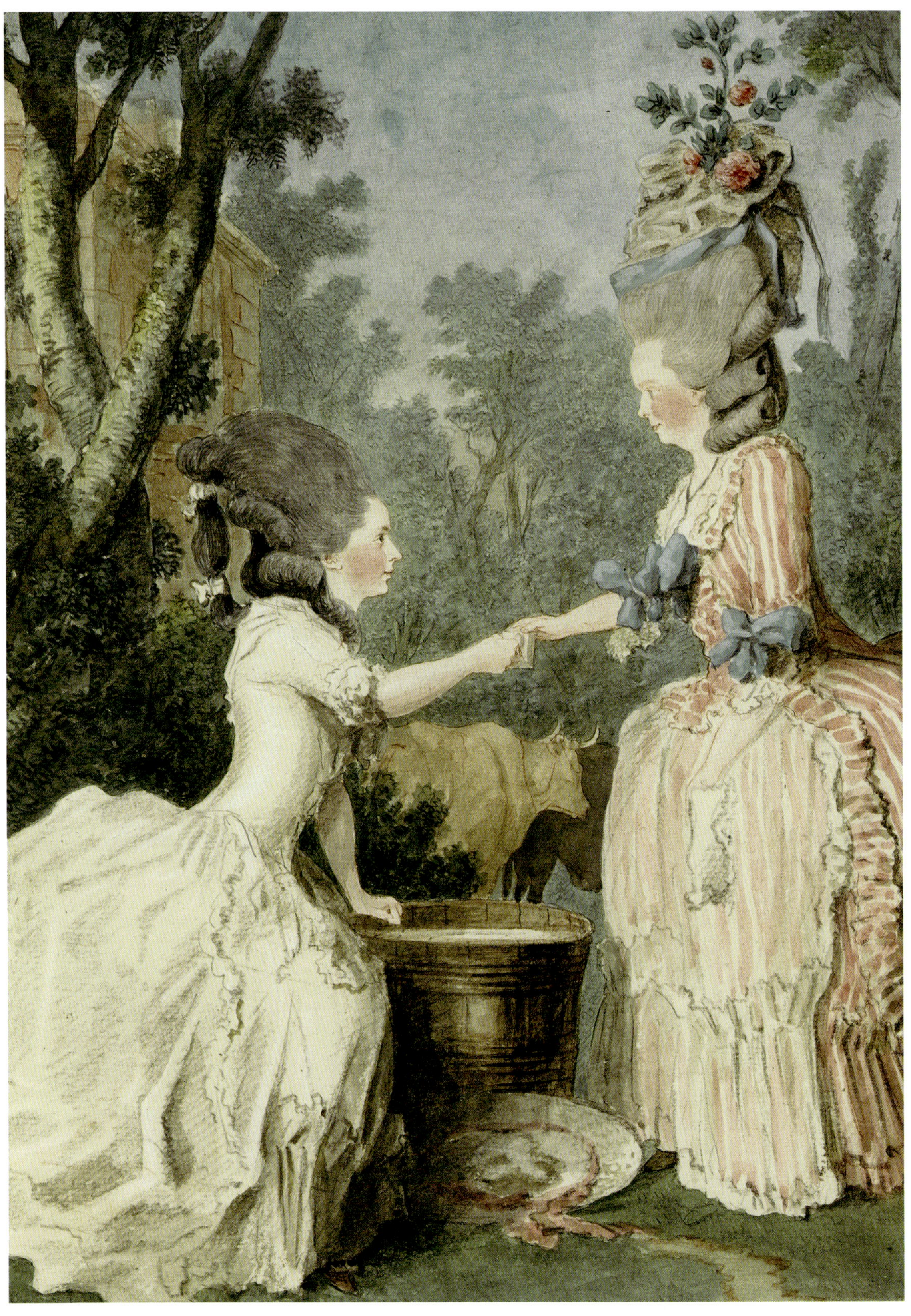

working so hard to sublimate or suppress. D'Angiviller had hoped that visitors would visit the Rambouillet dairy and be inspired by its message of royal rebirth, but by the time the dairy was finished in 1788, fewer of the crown's subjects were willing to regard the monarchy as redeemable or the queen as maternal rather than hopelessly dissolute. For her part, Marie-Antoinette preferred her pastoral retreat at Versailles, in whose gardens she was supposedly relaxing when she heard that an angry mob of citizens were planning to march on the palace in October 1789.

While the back-to-nature campaign contributed to a tragic demise for many aristocratic women, it had some undeniably comedic moments as well. Surely the most bizarre of the natural regimens invented in the eighteenth century to cure consumption, the vapors, and other urban illnesses was the "cow-house treatment." This method was popularized by the English physician Thomas Beddoes, whose target audience was, as he described them, "the ghastly beauties of the court and city," for whom "the ruddiness of the milk-maid has been a standing jest.'"[23] Beddoes recommended that such women take up residence in a cow stable for a goodly amount of time so that they could drink fresh milk, be surrounded by the comforting warmth of animals, and, above all, breathe in the curative fumes emitted by cow feces. Among those who attempted the regimen were the Princesse de Lamballe, a close friend of Marie-Antoinette, and Mrs. Sarah Finch, the daughter of the English scientist Joseph Priestley. Upon completing the treatment, the latter reported that though the stench made her "nauseous," it also improved her condition and made her "more than ever a friend to the cows."[24] Recognizing that not every patient was as game as Mrs. Finch, Beddoes came up with a less stringent version of the treatment that involved being confined to a heated apartment while vessels filled with cow shit were placed around the room. As far as I am aware, no eighteenth-century porcelain manufacturer designed a container for that.

1 Rosalind Savill, *The Wallace Collection Catalogue of Sèvres Porcelain*, vol. 2 (London: Trustees of the Wallace Collection, 1988), p. 668.
2 Robert Finlay, "The Pilgrim Art: The Culture of Porcelain in World History," *Journal of World History*, vol. 9, no. 2 (Fall 1998), p. 175.
3 I discuss the history of the milk cure in more detail in *Dairy Queens: The Politics of Pastoral Architecture from Catherine de' Medici to Marie-Antoinette* (Cambridge, Mass: Harvard University Press, 2011). Unless otherwise indicated, the material contained in this article, especially that related to the physicians, architectural sites, and women patrons discussed below, derives from this book.
4 William Coleman, "Health and Hygiene in the *Encyclopédie*: A Medical Doctrine for the Bourgeoisie," *Journal of the History of Medicine and Allied Sciences*, vol. 29, no. 4 (October 1974), p. 406.
5 Samuel Tissot, *De la santé des gens de lettres* [1768] (Geneva: Slatkine, 1981). See also Anne C. Vila, *Enlightenment and Pathology: Sensibility in the Literature and Medicine of Eighteenth-Century France* (Baltimore: Johns Hopkins University Press, 1998), pp. 187–196.
6 Jean-Jacques Rousseau, *Julie, ou La nouvelle Héloïse* [1761], trans. Philip Stewart and Jean Vaché (Hanover: Dartmouth College, 1997), p. 372.
7 Quoted from Venel's entry "Lait" in Denis Diderot and Jean Le Rond d'Alembert, eds., *Encyclopédie, ou Dictionnaire raisonné des sciences, des arts et des métiers* (Paris: Briasson, 1751–1765).
8 Jeremy D. Popkin, ed., *Panorama of Paris: Selections from* Le Tableau de Paris *by Louis-Sébastien Mercier* (University Park, Pa.: Pennsylvania State University Press, 1999), pp. 69, 141.
9 "Franchipane" and other lab-engineered milk extracts are discussed in Barbara Orland, "Enlightened Milk: Reshaping a Bodily Substance into a Chemical Object," in Ursula Klein and E. C. Spary, eds., *Materials and Expertise in Early Modern Europe: Between Market and Laboratory* (Chicago: University of Chicago Press, 2010), pp. 163–197.
10 Rosalind Savill reports that the term *trembleuse* was used in Sèvres records from 1767, 1773, and 1774. She also notes that socketed saucers were invented in 1759 and were "probably intended for the sick." See *The Wallace Collection Catalogue*, op. cit., pp. 674, 675.
11 Samuel Richardson, *Clarissa, or the History of a Young Lady* [1747–1748] (London: Penguin Books, 1998), p. 1008; *Pamela, or Virtue Rewarded* [1740] (London: Penguin Classics, 1985), p. 373.
12 Philippe Sylvestre Dufour, *Traitez nouveaux et curieux du café, du thé et du chocolate* (The Hague: Chez Adrian Moetjens, 1685). See also Christine Lahaussois, *Porcelaines de Saint-Cloud* (Paris: Réunion des musées nationaux, 1997).
13 Amanda Lange, "Chocolate Preparation and Serving Vessels in Early North America," in Louis E. Grivetti and Howard-Yana Shapiro, eds., *Chocolate: History, Culture, and Heritage* (Hoboken, NJ: John Wiley and Sons, Inc., 2009), p. 138.
14 Numerous examples of Du Paquier *trembleuses* are described and illustrated in Johann Kräftner, ed., *Baroque Luxury Porcelain: The Manufactories of Du Paquier in Vienna and of Carlo Ginori in Florence* (Vienna: Prestel, 2005).
15 Roy Porter, "Consumption: Disease of the Consumer Society?" in John Brewer and Roy Porter, eds., *Consumption and the World of Goods* (London: Routledge, 1993), p. 64. Porter uses the term "badge of gentility" to refer to a distinctively British form of nervous or consumptive illness that was dubbed "the English Malady."
16 See, for example, Pierre Hunauld, *Dissertation sur les vapeurs et les pertes de sang* (Paris: J.-N. Leloup, 1756), which claims that coffee and chocolate can exacerbate the symptoms of vaporous women. See p. 131.
17 Quesnay is better known as the co-founder of Physiocracy, the eighteenth-century economic theory that extolled land as the true source of a nation's vitality and health.
18 Rosalind Savill, *The Wallace Collection Catalogue*, op. cit., p. 675.
19 Louis de Carmontelle (Louis Carrogis), *La Rosière*, published in *Proverbes et comedies posthumes de Carmontel, précédés d'une notice par Madame de Genlis*, vol. 2 (Paris: Ladvocat, 1825).
20 These pre-Revolutionary pamphlets (including one entitled *Essai historique sur la vie de Marie-Antoinette d'Autriche*) began to circulate widely in 1789, when royal censorship laws were lifted. See Simon Burrows, *Blackmail, Scandal, and Revolution: London's French Libellistes, 1758–92* (Manchester: Manchester University Press, 2006), chapter 6. Her trial transcripts are reprinted in Gérard Walter, ed., *Procès de Marie-Antoinette* (Brussels: Éditions Complexe, 1993).
21 D. T. de Bienville, *La Nymphomanie ou traité de la fureur utérine* (Amsterdam: Marc-Michel Rey, 1771), pp. 99–124.
22 See the pamphlet *Les Fureurs utérines de Marie-Antoinette, femme de Louis XVI* (Paris, 1791).
23 Thomas Beddoes, *Manual of Health; or, The Invalid Conducted Safely Through the Seasons* (London: J. Johnson, 1806), p. 14, quoted in Roy Porter, "Reforming the Patient in the Age of Reform: Thomas Beddoes and Medical Practice," in Roger French and Andrew Wear, eds., *British Medicine in an Age of Reform* (London: Routledge, 1991), p. 20.
24 Quoted in Roy Porter, "Consumption: Disease of the Consumer Society?" op. cit., p. 70. See also Roy Porter, *Doctor of Society: Thomas Beddoes and the Sick Trade in Late-Enlightenment England* (London: Routledge, 1992).

TRAGIC CANDY, TIME
CAROL MAVOR

It is never a good thing to speak against *a little girl.*
—Roland Barthes, "Myth Today"

WONDERLAND IS IN THE AIR

It is 1957, the year Roland Barthes published *Mytholo-gies*. Audrey Hepburn has charmed her audiences with *Funny Face*. Barthes has described the film star in *Mythologies* as "woman as child, woman as kitten."[1]

In France and America, a girl sensation is erupting. The public has fallen in love with girls who are roughly 4,562.5 days old (12.5 years). And, for those less Humbert-Humbertish, there are child-women who are older, but somehow not. (Was Brigitte Bardot really so naive as to believe at age eighteen that mice laid eggs?)

"A breeze from Wonderland is in the air."[2] Girls are everywhere, not only in films, but also as authors. Just three years before, in 1954, the aggressive publisher René Julliard scored an international triumph with Fran-çoise Sagan's *Bonjour Tristesse*. Sagan was eighteen years old. (By 1957, the childish, boyish, sexy Jean Seberg will star in the film adaptation of *Bonjour Tristesse*.)

Just a year earlier, in 1956, Vladmir Nabokov had published *Lolita* and B.B. (Brigitte Bardot) found herself to be an American sensation for her role in *And God Created Woman*, where she childishly ate and made love with the "same unceremonious simplicity."[3] While the always-barefoot B.B. was preserving the "limpidity" of childhood *and* its "mystery,"[4] the aggressive Julliard scored again. After the success of *Bonjour Tristesse*, he snatched up the child-poet Minou Drouet and published her first book of poetry: *Arbre, mon ami* (Tree, My Friend). Drouet was only eight years old.

The familiar myth of the child (as innocent and as artistic genius) was ripened by Drouet. As James Kincaid has carefully schooled us: "We construct an emptiness, a child, and set it to dreaming."[5] Paradoxically, the empty innocence of Drouet (as the photographs proclaim) is sexual. Paradox, however, is not a contradiction: it is a rhetorical strategy, an artistic treatment of a logical problem. Myth itself, thereby, is a paradox: it cloaks truth in fiction and fiction in truth, as if it were a little girl.

The child is a studied myth; the girl is its most *pure* form.

In "Myth Today" (*Mythologies'* concluding essay), Barthes claims with witty Saussurean irony that this Lottelita, this Lolitchen, (think Nabokov and Werther), this poetess named Drouet, had her own system of signs. As Barthes explains with the clinical dis-

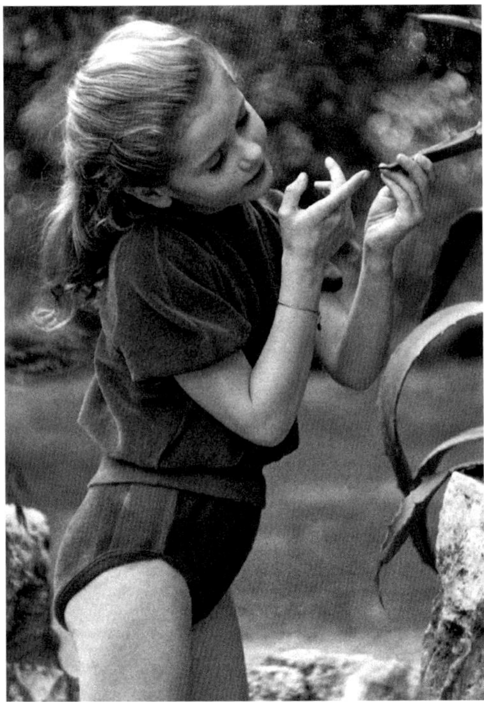

Minou Drouet, ca. 1956. A line from one her poems reads: "les cactus pour les touristes..." Photograph Roger Hauert.

interest of a scholar-man who likes boys, not girls: "A tree is a tree. Yes, of course. But a tree as expressed by Minou Drouet is no longer quite a tree, it is a tree which is decorated, adapted to a certain type of consumption, laden with literary self-indulgence, revolt, images, in short with a type of social *usage* which is added to pure matter."[6] Barthes's "semioclasm"[7] is out to destroy the "myth of Childhood-as-poet."[8]

In the French publication of *Mythologies*, the poetess gets an entire essay: "Literature According to Minou Drouet." There, Barthes further unveils Drouet's "nymphancy" as inseparable from her poetry.[9] But the little treatise was axed in 1972, when the book was translated into English. The famed Drouet had already been forgotten.

Today, as Robert Gottlieb notes, few people (especially those under a certain age) know much about Drouet, even in Paris. Was she a "victim" of her publisher? Did Cocteau say something "bitchy" about her?[10]

Who is Minou Drouet?

Today, she is Mme. Jean-Paul Le Canu. She is in her sixties. She lives in hibernation in her childhood home, under the shadow of the big cedar tree that she has always loved. It seems that she, too, has chosen to forget "la petite princesse des mots" (the little princess of words).[11]

Clock face,
crystal cage
        ...
siamese animal twin of my heart,
greedy eyes like children's eyes
who looking at pastries
undress the icing
from cakes all crackly with frost
mouth which nibbles with no respite
this tragic candy, time.
—Minou Drouet, "The Watch"

Once upon a time, in Brittany, Minou was born (1947). Minou means kitten (more accurately "pussy") in French. Her father was a very poor field hand. Many said that her mother was a prostitute. As we all know, in real life and in fairy tales, "daughters wander off into the woods, stumble into prostitution, fall in love with sailors, are eaten by wolves."[12] It was not such a promising beginning. But when she was a year-and-a-half old, a worrisome fairy godmother (and aspiring poetess) named Mme. Drouet adopted quiet, barely mewing Minou.

By age six, little Minou still had not spoken a word. She was tight-lipped and silent. Minou was Briar Rose waiting to be awakened. "Waiting is an enchantment."[13] ("Enfant. From the Latin *infans*; from *in* (not) and *fari* (to speak): the one who does not speak."[14])

"One day, her mother played a recording of a Brahms symphony for her. Minou swooned. When she was revived, she spoke perfect French in complex sentences. Shortly thereafter she began to write poetry."[15]

Minou had become enchanted.

Minou had become enchanting.

As in many fairy tales, Maman was the wicked stepmother. Mme. Drouet cracked the whip: ballet lessons, guitar lessons, hours of piano practice and gymnastics, "every minute accounted for."[16] Even though she could play Mozart while doing a backbend on the piano, Minou could never be perfect enough; one might even say "empty" enough. ("Innocence is ... like air ... there's not a lot you can do but lose it."[17]) Mme. Drouet beat the innocence (air) out of Minou for the most miniscule mistakes.

In a letter to the famous pianist Yves Nat, Minou complains:

Little girls' bottoms are really a wonderful gift
from heaven for calming the nerves of moth-
ers. I know perfectly well that's what they were

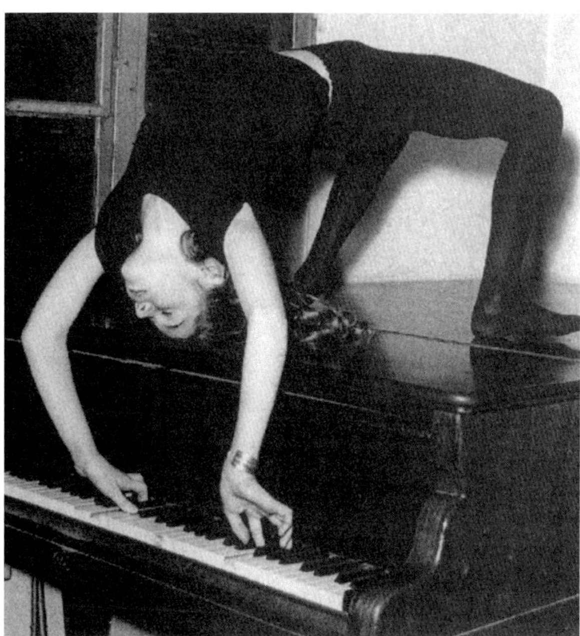

Drouet performing acrobatics while playing a sonata by Mozart, ca. 1960.

invented for, for hands have hollows and bottoms
have humps. It's because of you that I had my
bottom spanked, because I didn't write Mr. in the
address and didn't put a capital letter.[18]

Minou's letter smacks of Eve Kosofksy Sedgwick's girlhood poetry under the rap of spanking. As Sedgwick writes in her 1987 startling retelling of Freud's "A Child Is Being Beaten" as "A Poem is Being Written": "When I was a little child the two most rhythmic things that happened to me were spanking and poetry."[19] Sedgwick confesses that, as a girl, she took sexual pleasure in writing poetry with plenty enjambment to the eroticized beat of being spanked. (But for Sedgwick the results were much different.)

In the same letter, Minou speaks of "angry trees which seem to be kicking at the sky, trees through which something so gentle was passing."[20] Minou's words are strangely in accord with Hans Bellmer's 1935 photograph of Drouetish legs kicking their Mary Janes and bobby socks up into the trees.[21] The *poupée* legs (those standing and those kicking) are in bondage with, and/or in love with, these trees that grow in likeness with them. A shadowed figure lurks.

A strange and troubled child, Minou was odd. Minou did not fit in. As she writes in "Photograph," "I brought you nothing / but an ugly face / a nose for telephoning to the clouds ..."[22] Minou found solace in the tree that she loved, her true friend, who lived (and still

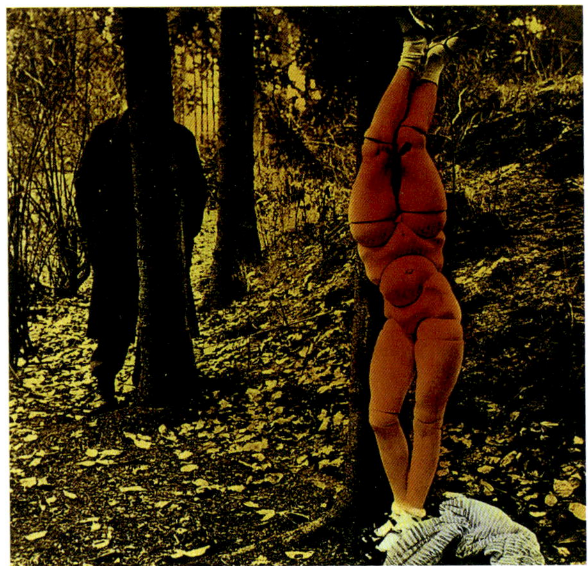

Hans Bellmer, *The Doll*, 1935.

does) in her garden in la Guerche de Bretagne, "a very big cedar of Lebanon."[23]

> *Tree that I love,*
> *tree in my likeness,*
> *so heavy with music*
> *under the wind's fingers*
> *that turn your pages*
> *like a fairy tale,*
> *tree …*[24]

Remember what Barthes says in "Myth Today": "A tree is a tree. Yes of course. But a tree as expressed by Minou Drouet is no longer quite a tree."[25]

SHE IS AN EIGHTY-YEAR-OLD DWARF

If a bit overly sweet, this little kitten's surrealist style was reminiscent of André Breton. But the public was suspicious of her "genius," and claimed her mother was the true author of Minou's disturbing, delicious, wild poems. Jean Cocteau, who made his own fairy-tale film of *Beauty and the Beast*, famously quipped: "She's not an eight-year-old child, she's an 80-year-old dwarf."[26] Cocteau saw her as Rumpelstiltskin, not Snow White.

It was in 1955, when some of Minou's poems and letters were privately circulated among French writers and publishers, that what Julliard called a "minor Dreyfus Affair" began. Almost overnight, there were appearances on television and articles in magazines and newspapers. People took sides. Did she write the

poems or not? Minou became a French and American sensation. Minou was photographed by *Elle*, *Life*, *Time*, and *Paris Match*: at her desk with her pen in hand, with her teddy bear, with her adoptive mother and cat, and almost always with that giant Drouet bow. (The bow is not only Bellmer's metonymy, it is also Minou's.)

On 20 January 1956, a test was organized by the Société des Auteurs (SACEM) to discover the truth: "Minou was placed in a room behind one-way glass."[27] She was told she could write on "I am Eight Years Old" or "Paris Sky." Since, as she claimed, her "eight years were already too sad," she chose "Paris Sky."[28] Within twenty-eight minutes she wrote "Ciel de Paris." It was written in the shape of Minou's beloved tree; like Apollinaire, she liked to make her poems into calligrammes, serpentine shapes, crystal cages of words.

> *Paris Sky,*
> *weight,*
> *secret,*
> *flesh,*
> *who by hiccups,*
> *spits in our faces*
> *through the open maw of rows of houses*
> *a spurt of blood*
> *between its luminous stumps of bad teeth …*[29]

Drouet is Shirley Temple on the good ship lollipop: swallowed by the mouth that hiccups and "spits in our faces" the myths of little girls as sugar and spice and everything nice. Drouet is Berenice trapped in Joseph Cornell's 1943 *The Crystal Cage*, like jelly in the sugary doughnuts that he childishly loved.

The SACEM test was a modern-day fairy tale: Drouet was Snow White in a glass box (coffin). Would she feel the pea under the pile of mattresses? Would her foot easily slip into the glass slipper?[30] As Barthes notes: it was "a detective story: did she do it or didn't she?"[31] (Fairy tales are always detective stories: they sort out real princesses from imposters.)

In the end, she won. She was awarded membership.

LET'S EAT HER

> *That young tender thing would be a delicious morsel.*
> —Brothers Grimm, "Little Red Cap"

> *My only grudge against nature was that I could*
> *not turn my Lolita inside out and apply voracious*
> *lips to her young matrix, her unknown heart, her*

*nacreous liver, the sea-grapes of her lungs, her
comely twin kidneys.*
—Vladimir Nabokov, *Lolita*

*I must be a little rabbit who once turned its fur
inside out for fear of moths.*
  —Minou Drouet, extract from a notebook

As markers of lost time, photographs are always-
already tragic, deadly murderers of life once lived,
perhaps especially if they are picturing a sweet little
girl like Drouet. The camera is a killing "mouth which
nibbles with no respite / this tragic candy, time."[32] Likewise, in *Camera Lucida*, Barthes glazes the photograph
as sugar housed in the violence that originally bespoke
the fairy tale:

*The Photograph is violent: not because it shows
violent things, but because on each occasion it
fills the sight by force, and because in it nothing
can be refused or transformed (that we can sometimes call it mild does not contradict its violence:
many say that sugar is mild, but to me sugar is violent, and I call it so).*[33]

The photograph, then, is brutal not only like sugar,
but also like Perrault's original fairy tales, in which the
eyes of Cinderella's sisters are pecked out and Hansel
and Gretel are almost eaten.

The large letter *O*, which begins fairy tales with
great ornamental flurry, is derived from the Egyptian
hieroglyph for the eye: both the iris and the pupil are
circles. Yet an *O* is also an open mouth. The eye and the
mouth ingest as figures of *oralia*.[34] (*O* is also for *oralia*.)
While *oralia* emphasizes the double consumption of
the mouth as eye, it is also a variant of the Latin *aurelia*,
which means "golden." When Bellmer (in another doll
photograph, this one from 1934) places a headless
poupée on a large letter *O* crowned with a bow, with
her eye spit back onto her footless ankle, the emptiness
of the child is perversely set to dreaming. It is the start
of a surreal Once-upon-a-time tale that is not so far from
the (un)golden childhood that was lived by Minou.

Barthes does not like "Drouetist poetry."[35] It is
"docile, sugary poetry,"[36] "stuffed" with "formulas."[37]
According to Barthes, Drouet fulfills a cultural desire to
demote and to tame literature into a sweet nothing.

As Richard Howard notes: "In the central range of
French language, there is no word for child … If there
have been children in French Literature, they are there
as mere instances of acculturation; as victims (Hugo,

Joseph Cornell, *The Crystal Cage (Portrait of Berenice)*, 1943.

Renard), as cult objects (Hugo again, Gide); either assimilated by Society as in infants (speechless) or transformed into members (remembered) or extruded as freaks (Minou Drouet)."[38]

As Barthes writes: "She is the kidnap victim of a conformist order which reduces freedom to prodigy status. She is the little girl the beggar pushes onto the sidewalk when back home the mattress is stuffed with money."[39] Through Minou's own delectably violent words, we look at her with "greedy eye like children's eyes / who looking at pastries / undress the icing / from cakes all crackly with frost / mouth which nibbles with no respite / this tragic candy, time."[40]

Barthes is anorexic when it comes to eating Drouet. "It may happen that I feel no hunger for the world," claims Barthes in *The Neutral*, "but the world will force me to love it, to eat it, to enter into intercourse with it."[41] Barthes tells us that "society is devouring Minou Drouet,"[42] but he remains tight-lipped, refusing to partake in "this tragic candy."

Completely sugarcoated and consumed by the time she was fourteen, Minou lost her passionate desire to write.

As in the years before she was six, Minou is once again silent. She is back to sleep, forever held as the bowed, Bellmeresque little girl of "tragic candy, time," with no hope of being de-windowed ("dévitriné"),[43] of escaping her crystal cage, her glass coffin. Forever and ever, she is stuck as a little girl in the glass-covered daguerreotype of her eight-year-old self.

I look at a photograph of Minou at age eight and I "shudder" at the loss of this little girl. As Barthes writes about the Winter Garden Photograph (which captured his mother as a little girl): "I shudder [*je frémis*] like Winnicott's psychotic patient, *over a catastrophe which has already occurred*." (In English, *shudder* is a homonym for *shutter*.)

1 Roland Barthes, "Myth Today," in *Mythologies*, selected and translated by Annette Lavers (New York: Hill and Wang, 1972), p. 57. First published in French as *Mythologies* (Paris: Editions du Seuil, 1957).

2 Vladmir Nabokov, *The Annotated Lolita*, ed. Alfred Appel, Jr. (New York: McGraw-Hill, 1977), p. 133.

3 Simone de Beauvoir, "Brigitte Bardot and the Lolita Syndrome" [1959], in Elizabeth Sussman and Sidra Stich, eds., *Rosemarie Trockel* (New York: Prestel, 1991), p. 55.

4 Simone de Beauvoir, op. cit., p. 54.

5 James Kincaid, "Dreaming the Past," paper presented at the University of North Carolina, Chapel Hill, 24 April 1993.

6 Roland Barthes, "Myth Today," op. cit., p. 109.

7 Roland Barthes, "Preface to the 1970 edition," *Mythologies*, op. cit., p. 9.

8 Roland Barthes, "Myth Today," op. cit., p. 149.

9 The term *nymphancy* is Nabokov's as used in *Lolita*, p. 224.

10 Robert Gottlieb, "A Lost Child: The Strange Case of Minou Drouet," *The New Yorker*, 6 November 2006, p. 70.

11 Jean-Max Tixier, "Notes," in Minou Drouet, *Ma vérité* (Paris: Editions 1, 1993), p. 14.

12 Sarah Sun-Lien Bynum, *Madeleine Is Sleeping* (New York: Harcourt, 2004), p. 72.

13 Roland Barthes, *A Lover's Discourse: Fragments*, trans. Richard Howard (New York: Hill and Wang, 1978), p. 38. First published in French as *Fragments d'un discours amoureux* (Paris: Editions du Seuil, 1977).

14 Richard Howard, "Childhood Amnesia," in *Yale French Studies*, no. 43 (1969), p. 165.

15 Charles Templeton, *An Anecdotal Memoir* (Toronto: McClelland and Stewart Limited: The Canadian Publishers, 1983), p. 111.

16 Robert Gottlieb, "A Lost Child," op. cit., p. 73.

17 James Kincaid, *Erotic Innocence* (Durham, N.C.: Duke University Press, 2000), p. 53.

18 Minou Drouet to Yves Nat, letter in *First Poems*, trans. Margaret Crossland (London: Hamish Hamilton, 1956), p. 67.

19 Eve Kosofsky Sedgwick, "A Poem Is Being Written," in *Tendencies* (Durham, N.C.: Duke University Press, 1993), p. 182.

20 Drouet to Nat, op. cit., p. 67.

21 Bellmer took the picture in 1935 and then had it hand-colored in 1949. See Sue Taylor, *The Anatomy of Anxiety* (Cambridge, Mass: MIT Press, 2002), pp. 78, 204.

22 Minou Drouet, "Photographie," in *Le Pêcheur de lune* (Paris: Editions Pierre Horay, 1959), p. 79. ("*Je ne vous avais apporté / qu'un si laid visage, / un nez pour téléphoner / aux nuages ...*"). Translation mine.

23 Robert Gottlieb, "A Lost Child," op. cit., p. 76.

24 Minou Drouet, "Tree that I Love," in *First Poems*, op. cit., p. 3.

25 Roland Barthes, "Myth Today," op. cit., p. 109.

26 "Kitten on the Keys," *Time Magazine*, 28 January 1957.

27 Charles Templeton, *An Anecdotal Memoir*, op. cit., p. 112.

28 Robert Gottlieb, "A Lost Child," op. cit., p. 72.

29 Minou Drouet, "Ciel de Paris," in *Le Pêcheur de lune*, op. cit., p. 27. ("*Ciel de Paris, / poids, / secret, / chair, / qui, par hoquets, / crache à nos faces / par la gueule ouverte des rangées de maisons / un jet de sang entre ses chicots lumineux...*") Translation mine.

30 The glass slipper is Disney's addition. In the original fairy tale, the wicked sisters lop off heels and toes in order to squeeze into the slipper. However, given that Disney's *Cinderella* was produced in 1950, it does make a snug fit with Drouet.

31 Roland Barthes, "Literature According to Minou Drouet," trans. Richard Howard, in *Eiffel Tower and Other Mythologies* (Berkeley: University of California Press, 1979), p. 111. As stated, the essay was cut from the English edition of *Mythologies*, but it does reappear here in this collection of translated essays.

32 Minou Drouet, "The Watch," in *Then There Was Fire: Further Poems by Minou Drouet* (London: Hamish Hamilton, 1957), p. 32.

33 Roland Barthes, *Camera Lucida: Reflections on Photography*, trans. Richard Howard (New York: Hill and Wang, 1981), p. 91. First published in French as *La Chambre claire: Note sur la photographie* (Paris: Editions du Seuil, 1980).

34 Michael Moon, *A Small Boy and Others: Imitation and Initiation in American Culture from Henry James to Andy Warhol* (Durham, N.C.: Duke University Press, 1998), p. 138.

35 Roland Barthes, "Literature According to Minou Drouet," op. cit., p. 112.

36 Ibid., p. 114.

37 Ibid., p. 116.

38 Richard Howard, "Childhood Amnesia," op. cit., p. 166.

39 Roland Barthes, "Literature According to Minou Drouet," op. cit., p. 118.

40 Minou Drouet, "The Watch," op. cit., p. 32.

41 Roland Barthes, *The Neutral: Lecture Course at the Collège de France (1977–78)*, trans. Rosalind Krauss and Denis Hollier (New York: Columbia University Press, 2005), p. 153. First published in French as *Le Neutre* (Paris: Editions du Seuil, 2002).

42 Roland Barthes, "Literature According to Minou Drouet," op. cit., p. 118.

43 Barthes uses this term in another context to describe Bernard Faucon's photographs of mannequins, who appear to have been awakened, as if they escaped the department store window. See Barthes's "Bernard Faucon" in *Oeuvres complètes, Tome V, 1977–80*, ed. Éric Marty (Paris: Editions du Seuil, 2002), p. 472. First published in *Zoom*, 1978.

The convention of celebrating anniversaries with gifts of precious metals goes back to Central Europe in the Middle Ages, when tradition held that husbands would present their wives with first silver and then gold garlands to mark twenty-five and fifty years together, respectively. But it wasn't until the late nineteenth century that the vogue for recognizing each of the first ten anniversaries with a gift made from a particular material emerged in earnest, a developing custom that not surprisingly piqued the interest of business organizations like the American National Retail Jeweler Association. In 1937, the group published the list we used to commission the portfolio of projects on the following pages, created by some of our favorite artists to help celebrate *Cabinet*'s, ahem, own ten-year anniversary.

First Anniversary: Paper
Jane South, *Photographed, Printed, Copied, Faxed, Scanned, Published*, 2010.

Second Anniversary: Cotton
Ester Partegàs, *Obey Cosmic Wonder*, 2010.

Third Anniversary: Leather
Janine Antoni, *Perfect Bound (Editor-in-Chief)*, 2010.

Fourth Anniversary: Fruit
Rachel Harrison, *Balducci's*, 2010.

Fifth Anniversary: Wood
Francis Cape, *Untitled*, 2010.

Sixth Anniversary: Iron
Moyra Davey, *Tempus Fugit*, 2010.

Seventh Anniversary: Wool
Sabrina Gschwandtner, *Cabinet Cardigan*, 2010.
(knitted by Lindsay Degen)

Eighth Anniversary: Bronze
Alexandre Singh, *The Rotting Flesh*, 2010.

Ninth Anniversary: Pottery
Virgil Marti, *Untitled*, 2010.

Tenth Anniversary: Tin
Vik Muniz, *Cabinet of Curiosities*, 2010.

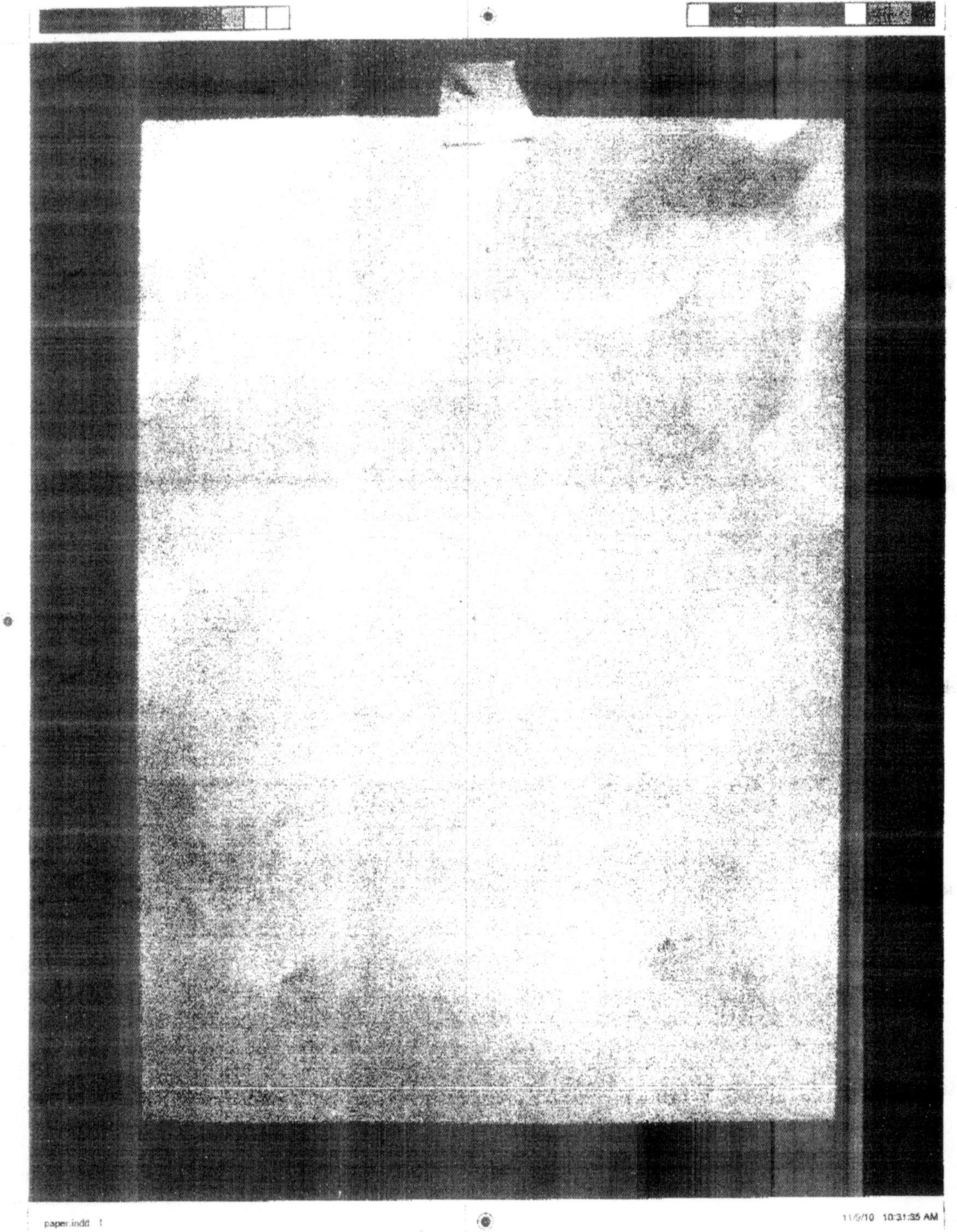

TOTAL PAGE(S) 01

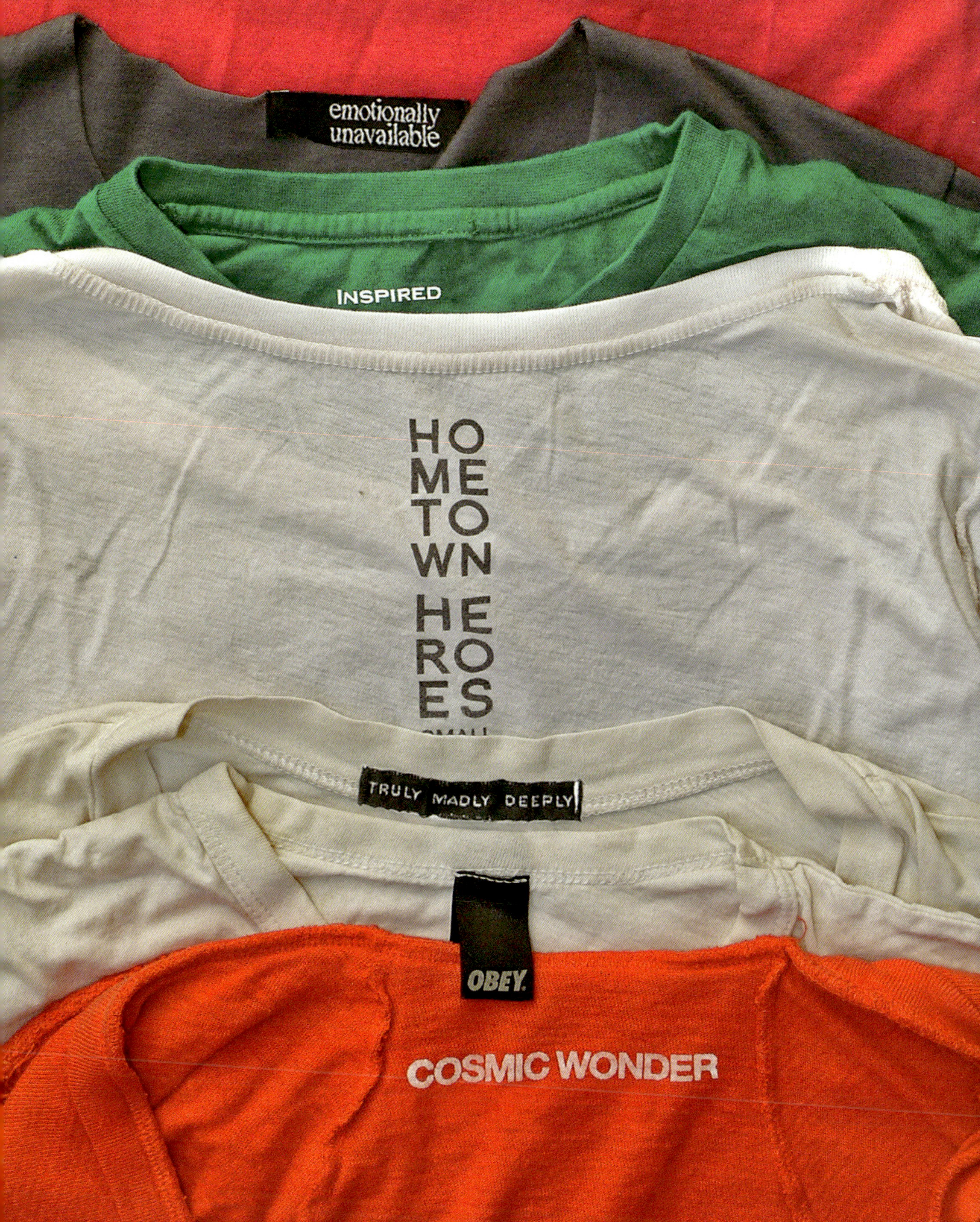

emotionally
unavailable
INSPIRED
HO
ME
TO
WN
HE
RO
ES
TRULY MADLY DEEPLY
OBEY.
COSMIC WONDER

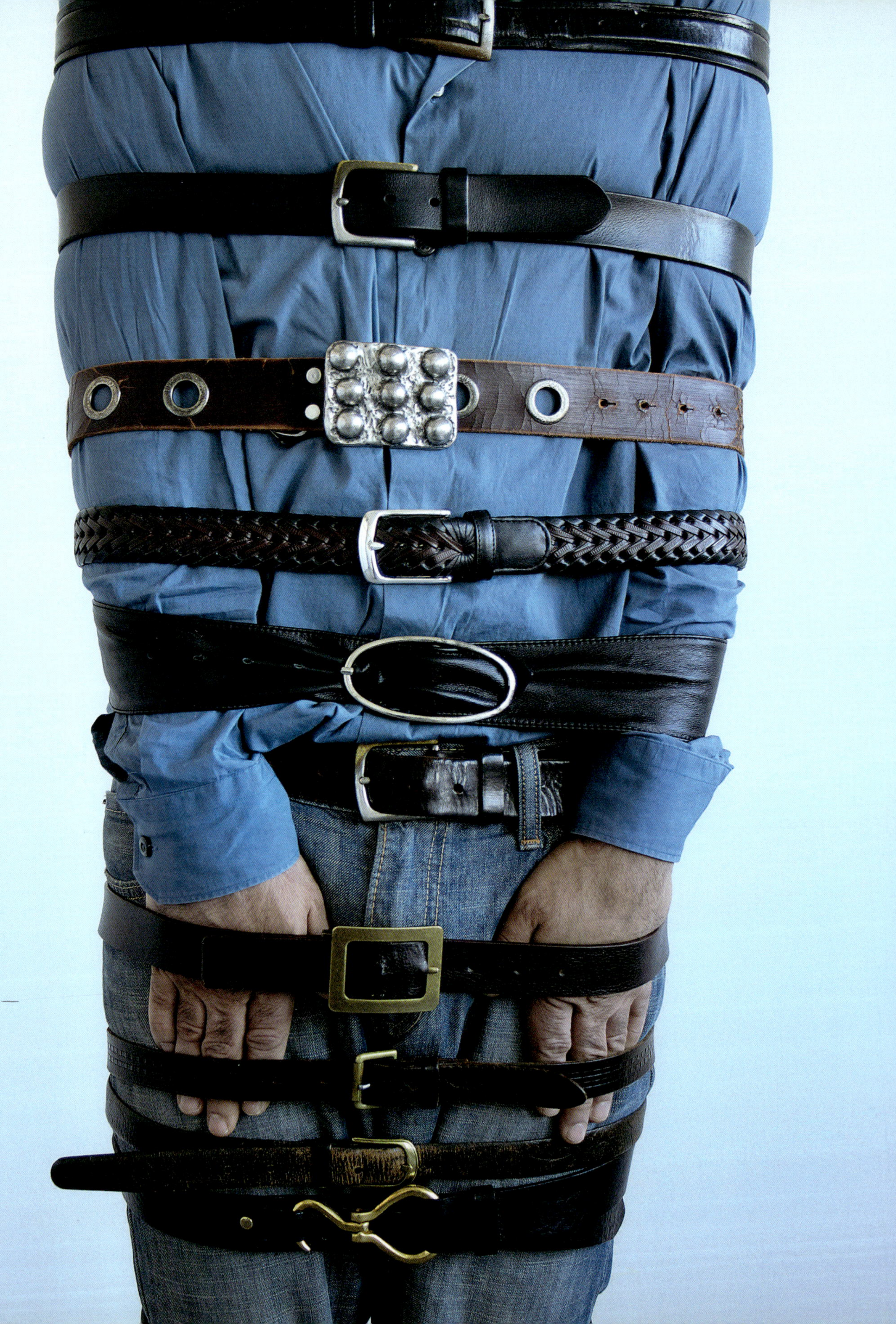

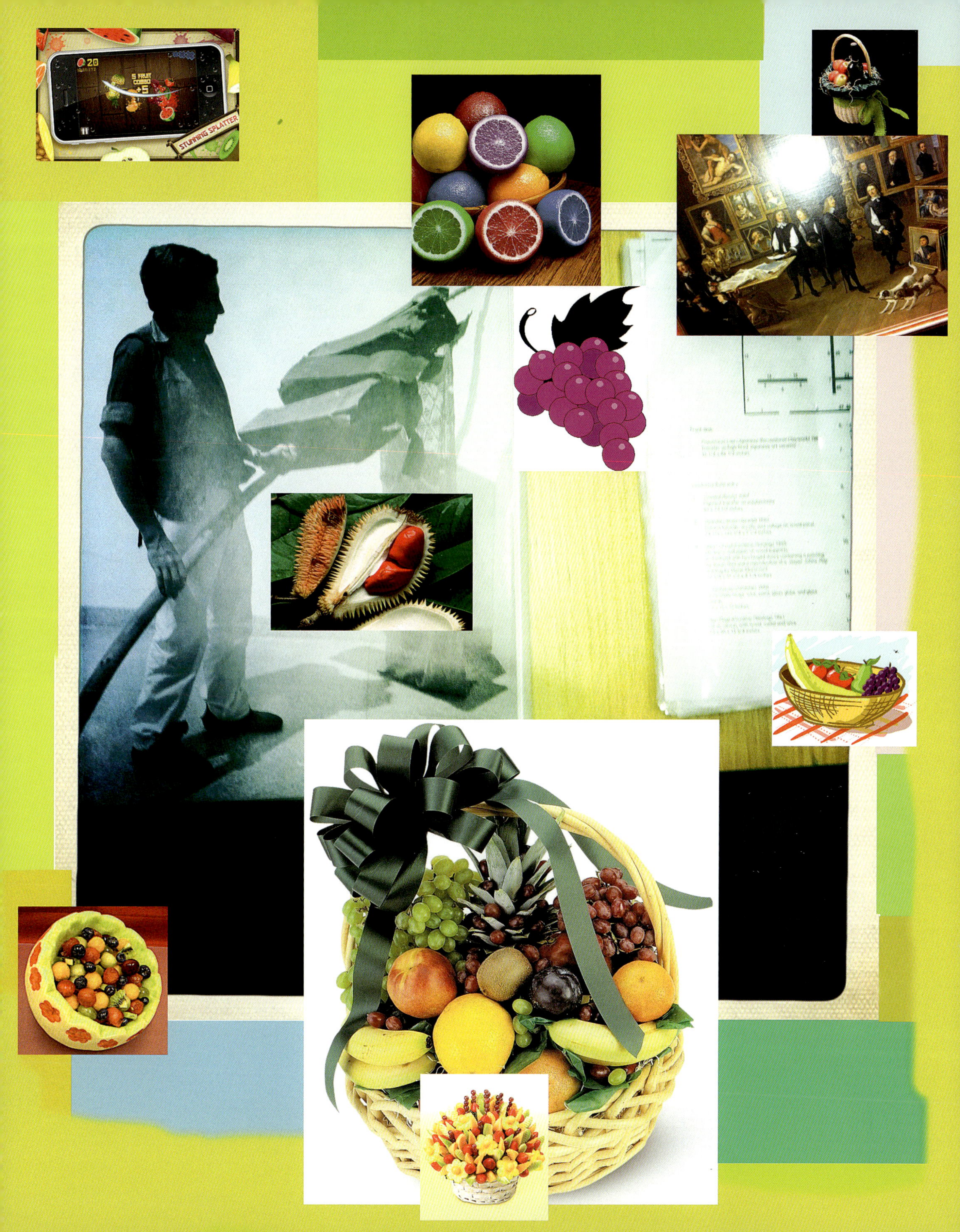

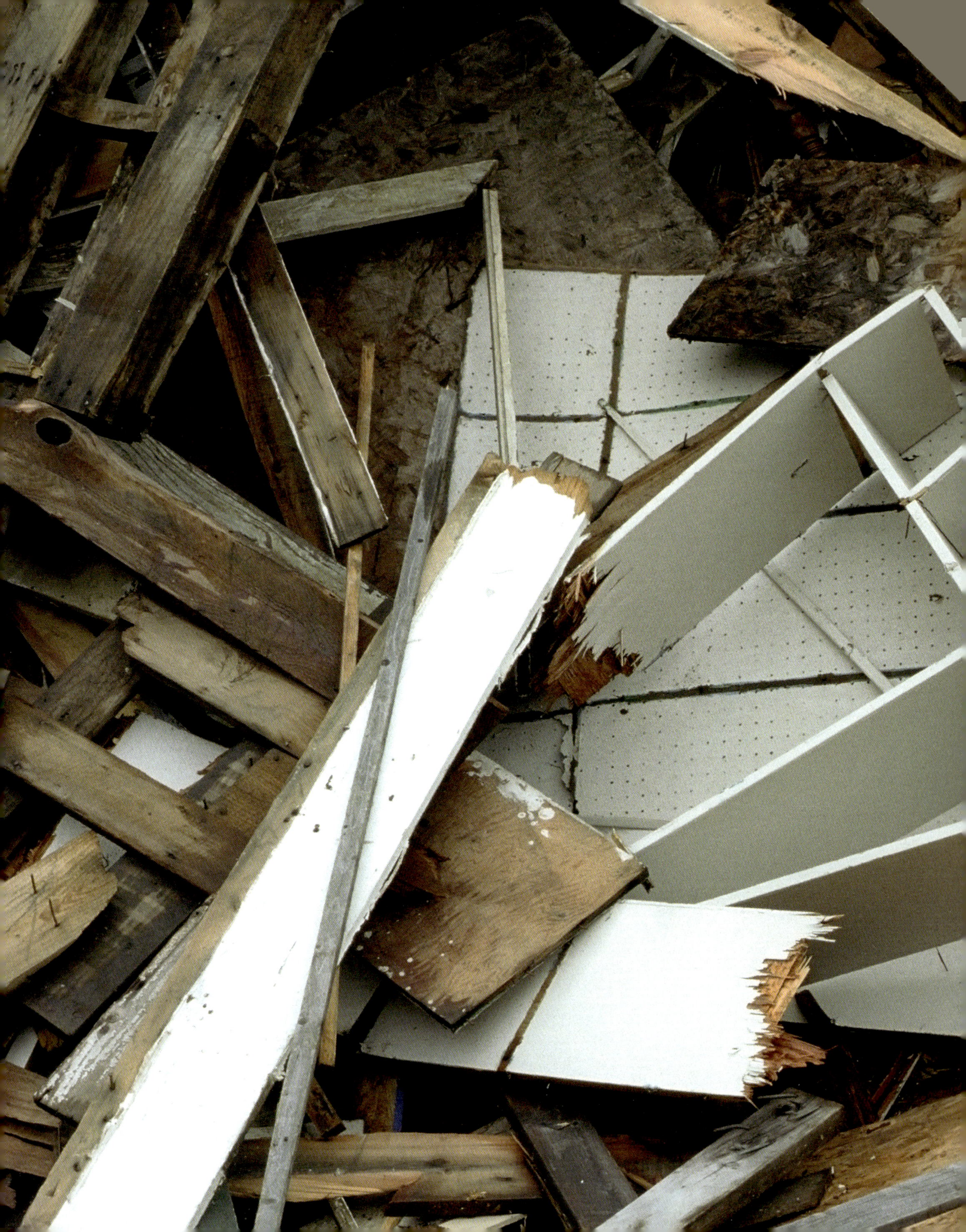

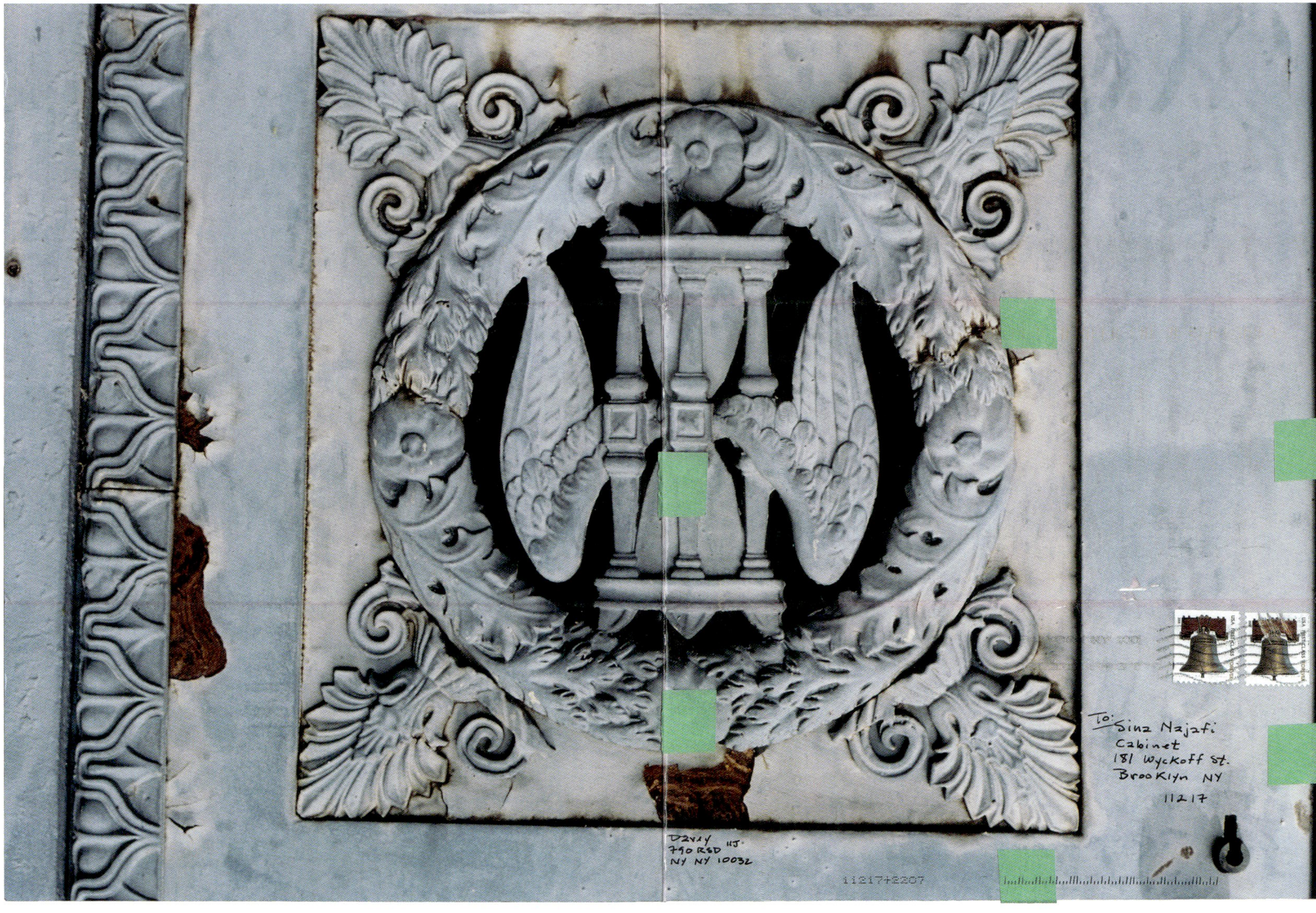
To: Sina Najafi
Cabinet
181 Wyckoff St.
Brooklyn NY
11217

Danny HS
740 RED ST
NY NY 10032

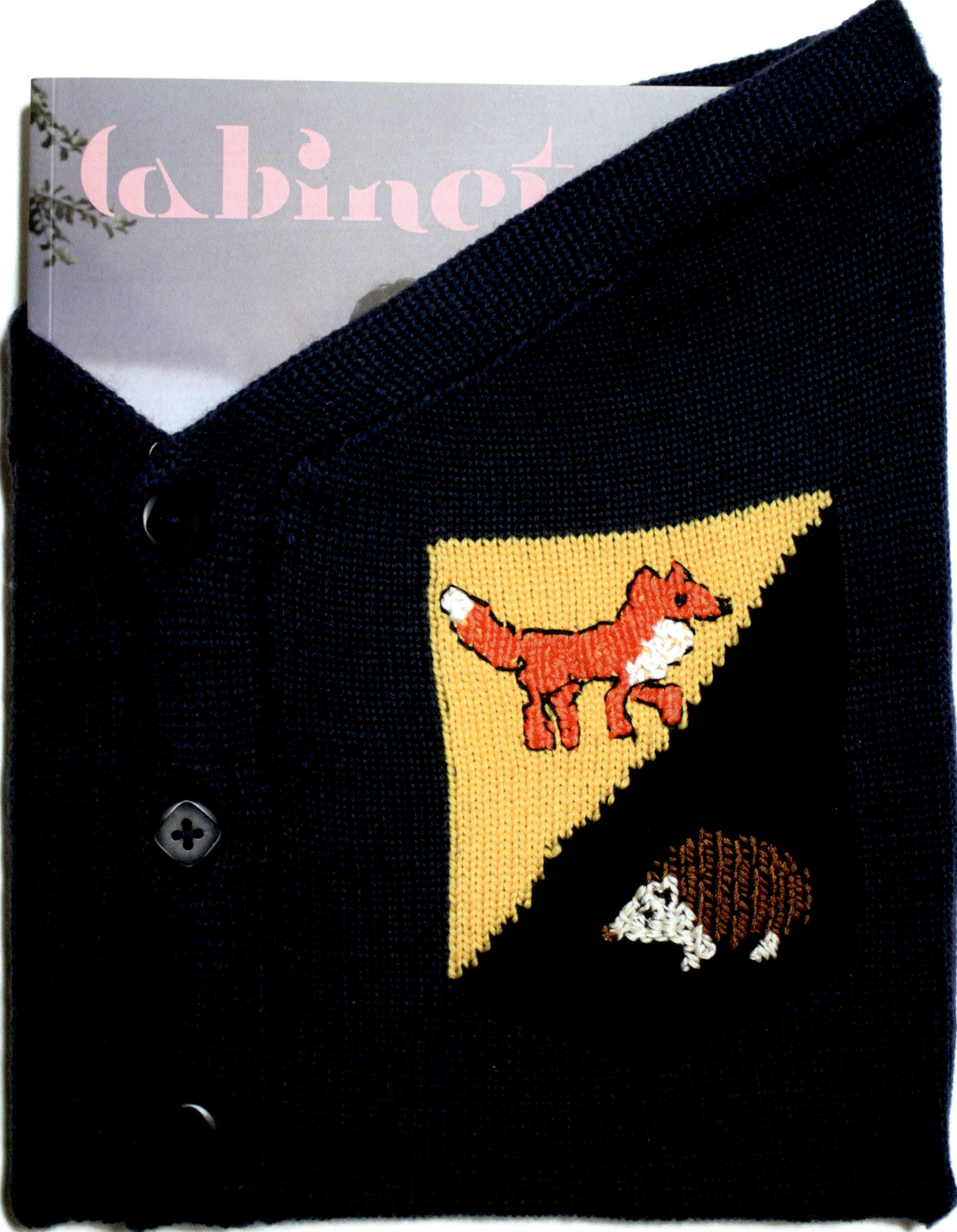

Cabinet

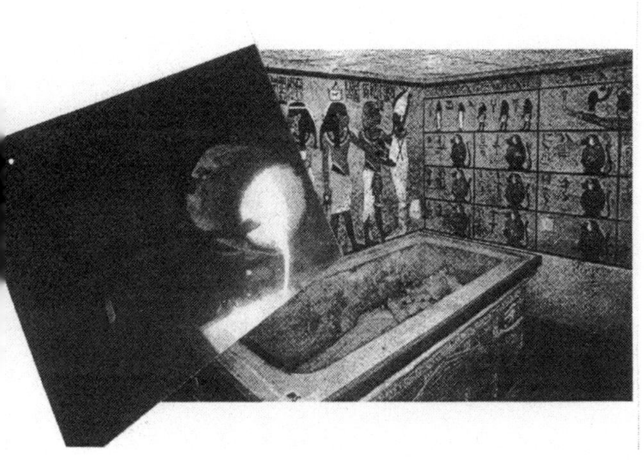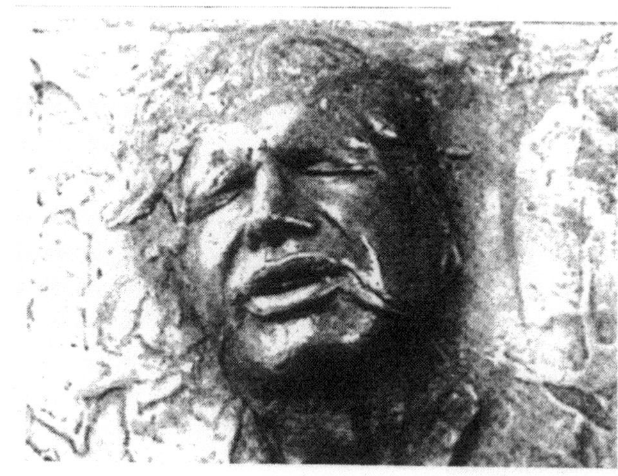

DIPPED IN BRONZE
THE ROTTING
FLESH
BENEVOLENTY
GAZES UPON THE
CITIZENRY URBAN
AND tourists.

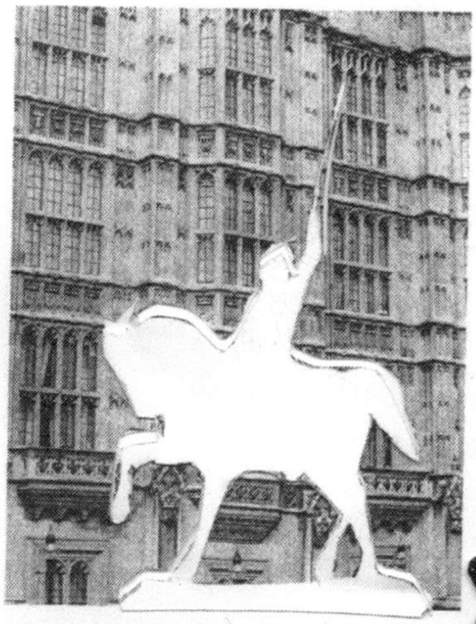

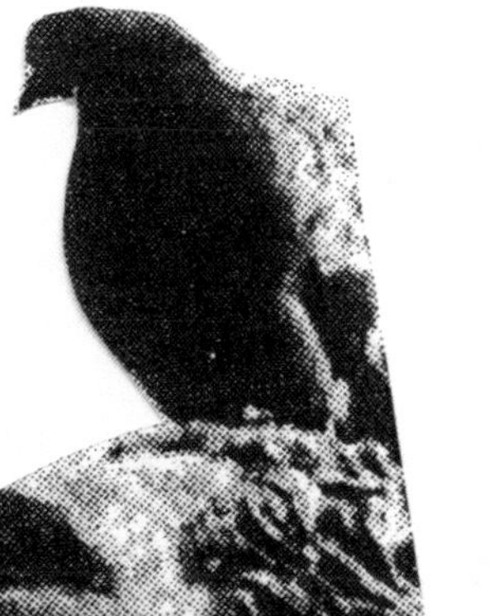

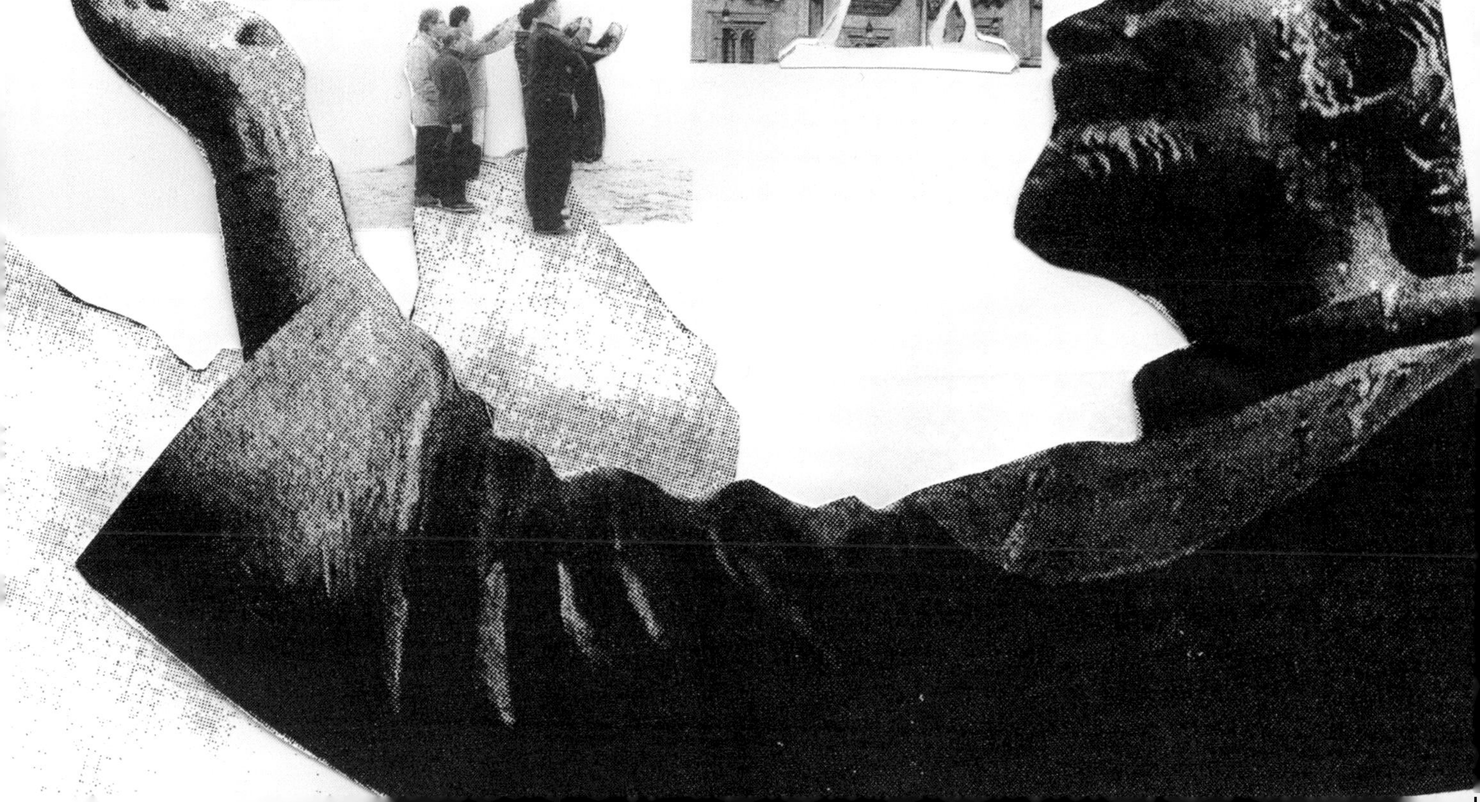

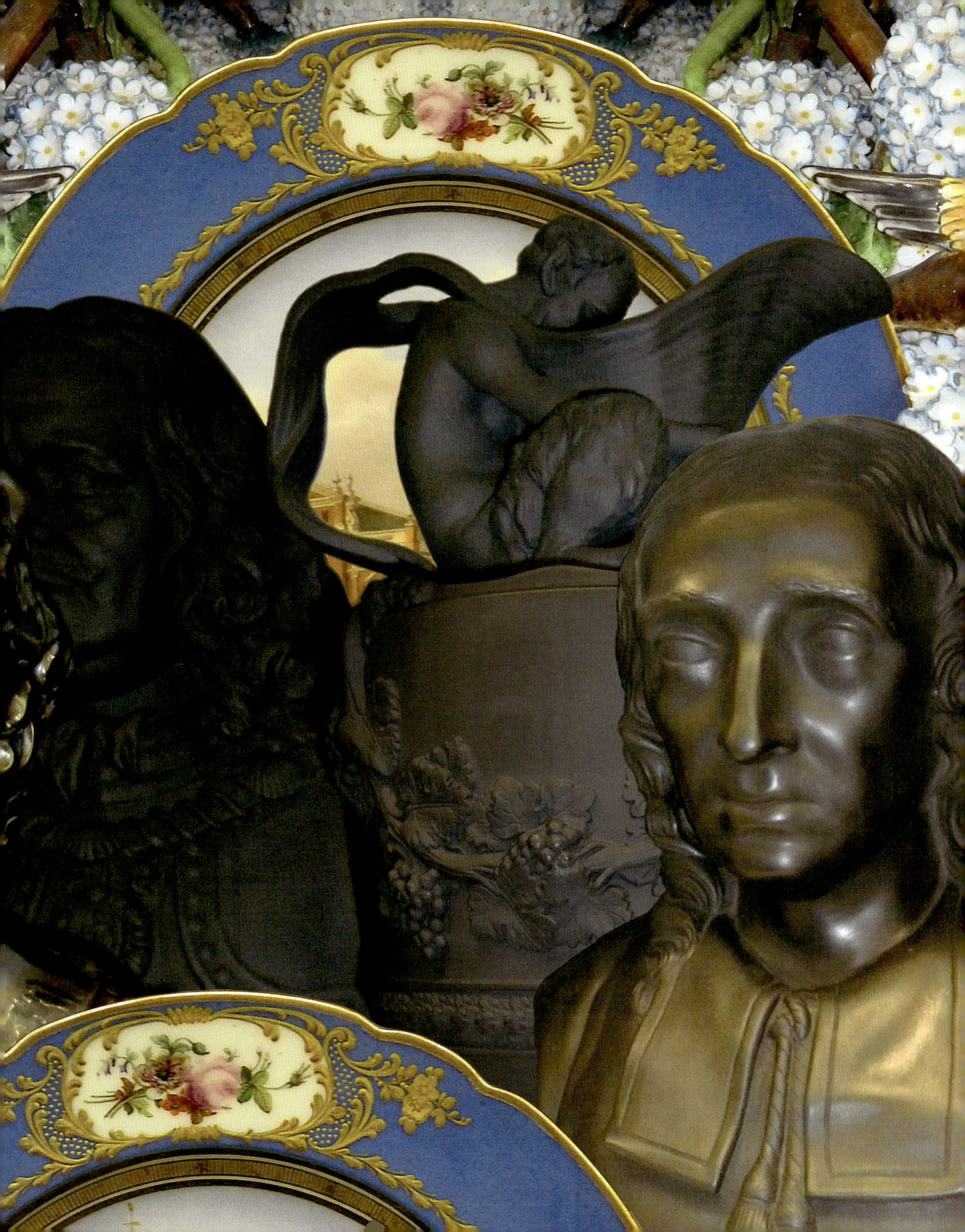

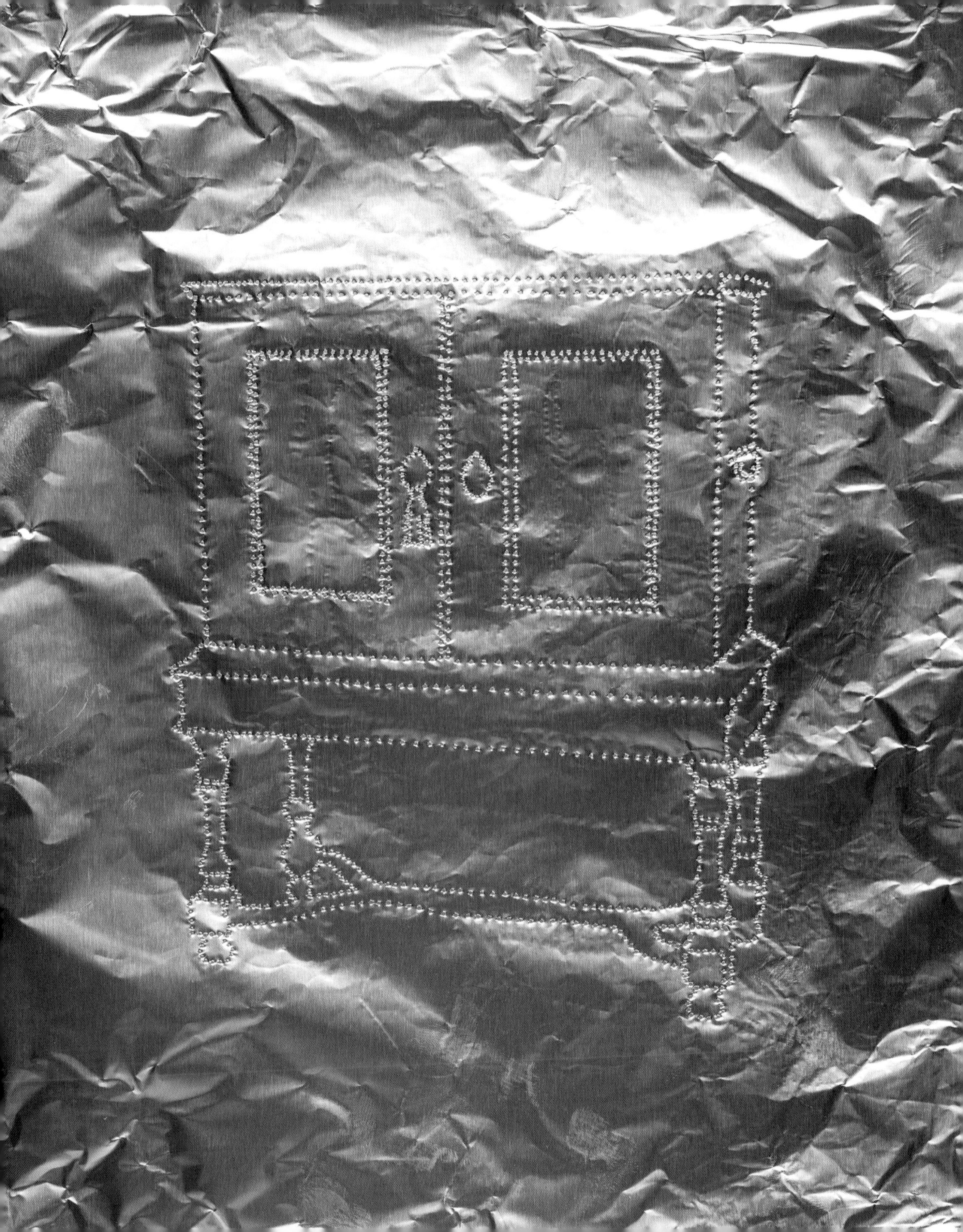

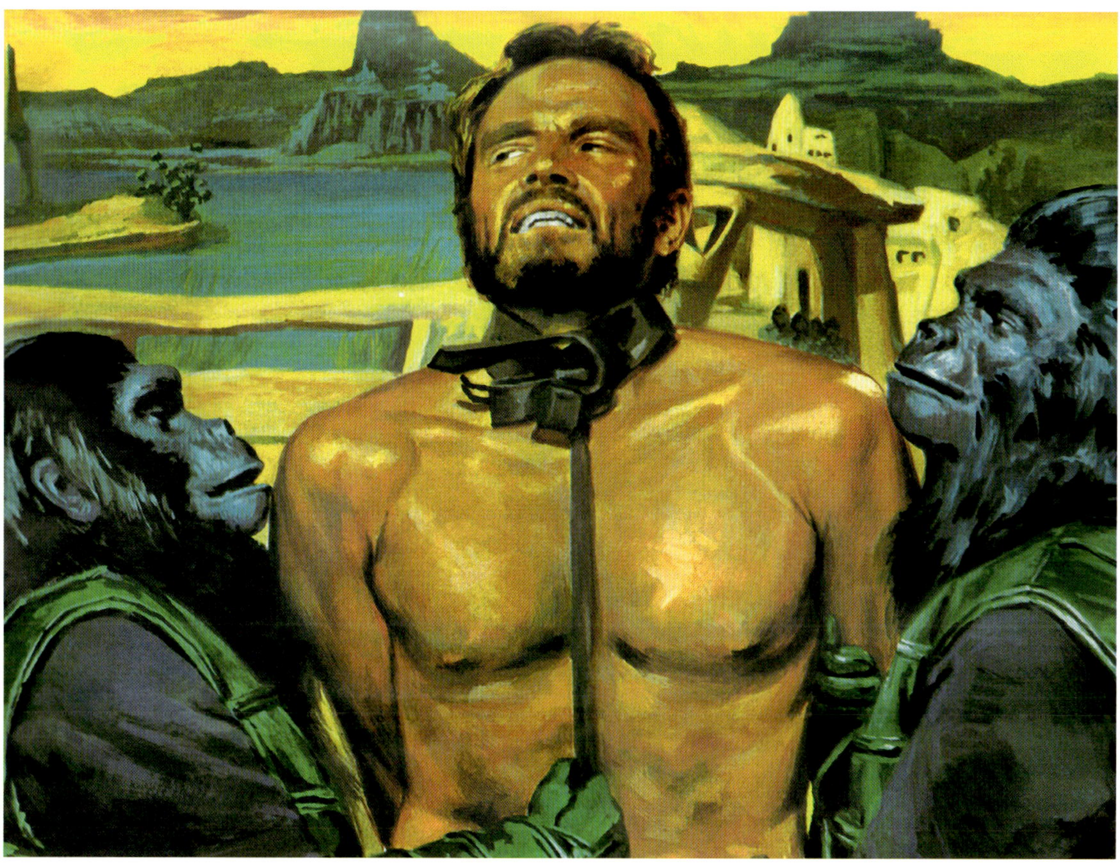

Hair as marker of civilization. Poster for 1970s French re-release of the 1968 film *Planet of the Apes*, starring Charlton Heston.

PATTERN BALDNESS

JUSTIN E. H. SMITH

It should come as no news here that hair is not only "for protection," as the deadpan evolutionary biologists tell us, but also for the differentiation of social roles, for the signalling of sexual availability, of political extremism, of class status, and of relative degrees of otherworldliness. Plato would judge hair too undignified to deserve an eternal, immutable Form of its own, yet what does the unkempt beard of a monk or a mullah signify if not his proximity to God?

For a time, in youth, the hair of the head may be manipulated into strange patterns, which signal subcultural belonging and so define the possible range of sex partners. The mohawk, the mullet, and the hi-top fade, no less than acne and the freshly sprouted pubic grove (protection from what, exactly?), are all just so many secondary sex characteristics, appearing with a bang that also announces the end of the dreamlike idyll of childhood.

But then, in males, the hairline often retreats, and the range of possible pompadours shrinks right along with the range of possible romantic pursuits. From Leviticus 13: 41–45 we learn of male pattern baldness: "He that hath his hair fallen off from the part of his head toward his face, he is forehead bald: yet is he clean." If, by contrast, "there be in the bald head a white reddish sore; it is a leprosy sprung up in his bald head, or his bald forehead," in which case "the priest shall pronounce him utterly unclean" since "his plague is in his head." Freedom from leprosy is nice enough, but what the forehead-bald man really wants is not to be clean but to be attractive, and it is no consolation that it was testosterone that causes the pattern baldness in the first place. This is semiotics, not endocrinology.

Anyway, the beard, which does not retreat but only grows thicker with age, says: to hell with all of this. I am old now and have no need for the games of youth. The seventeenth-century Baconian natural philosopher John Bulwer (also the inventor of sign language)

71

described it as the "naturall ensigne of Manhood appearing about the mouth." In his *Anthropometamorphosis, or the artificiall Changling* of 1650, he berated the "gallantry" and "foolish bravery" of those societies that permit their men to shave, since to do so is to hubristically interrupt with artifice the ordinary course of nature. He would not extend this prohibition to the fingernails, however, and even argued from scriptural evidence that Adam instinctively kept his nails groomed by biting them. Surely not the greatest inconsistency in the history of philosophy, but still, one does not have to strain to see that Bulwer was allowing his cultural norms to determine the boundaries of the natural.

Jump ahead to 1968, and you'll find Charlton Heston shaving on the beach, explaining to a talking ape from the future that, where he comes from, it is only the rebellious youth who let the ensigne of their manhood show about their mouths. The ape's response? But without it you look so *uncivilized*.

In all of this back-and-forth, in our various rearrangements of the patterns of hair and baldness, in our attentive reading of the different subtle signals of one another's *tomentum*, we are enabled to hold at bay, most of the time, any thought of what a strange thing it is to not be entirely covered with hair in the first place. With scattered exceptions (elephants, naked mole rats), hairlessness is a most peculiar thing among terrestrial mammals, and it is not hard to imagine other creatures looking at us the way we look at sphynx cats: as perversions of the ordinary course of things. Yet so prideful are we that we instead take this unusual feature as another sign, along with bipedality and rationality, that we are not really animals at all.

Of course, nothing is without a cause, and whatever it was that made us hairless, it was not some majestic transcendence of the animal condition. The precise evolutionary forces in play are, however, still a matter of some controversy. Elaine Morgan's so-called Aquatic Ape Hypothesis (AAH) has failed to gain much traction in the scientific establishment, perhaps because it is faulty, perhaps because she herself is not a member of that establishment. In her view, the ancestors of humans were beach-dwelling, quasi-marine mammals. Morgan believes that there is a convergence of facts supporting this account: for example, the diets of human beings require fatty acids most readily available in seafood; humans tend to have an unusually thick layer of insulating adipose cells, and so on. But the key bit of evidence, on this hypothesis, is that we are hairless.

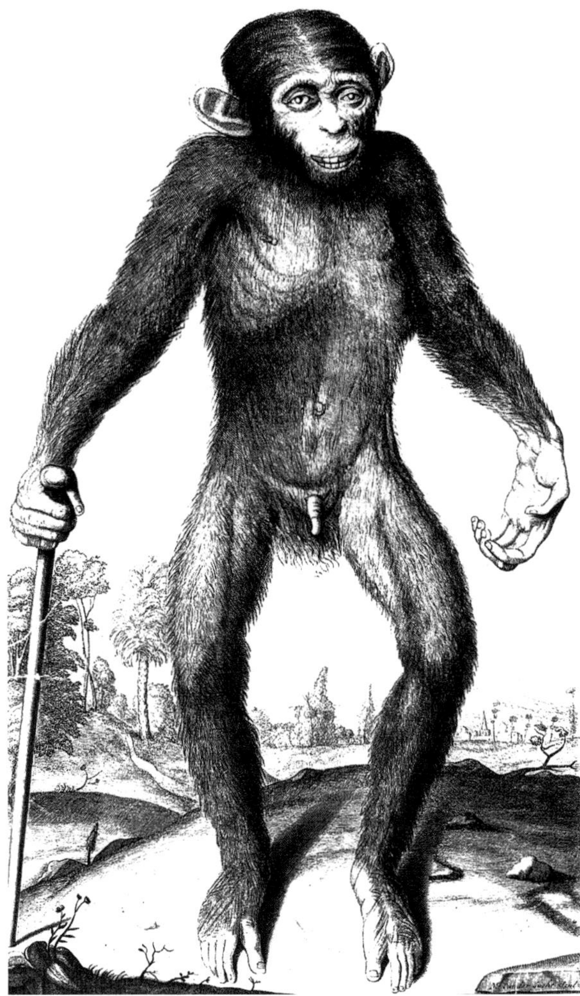

Edward Tyson's "orang-outang," in reality a chimpanzee. From Tyson's 1699 study *Orang-Outang sive homo silvestris*. Courtesy Wellcome Library.

In traditional terms, Morgan's hypothesis would make us even more perverse than one might have thought. In fact, it was not until recently that humans (literate, European humans, to be precise) began to accept that they had any business near water at all. Thomas Browne argued in his 1658 *Pseudodoxia epidemica*, a compendium of the false beliefs plaguing his era, that, plainly, swimming cannot be natural for men, since properly amphibious creatures "swim in the same manner as they go," needing "no other way of motion for natation in the water, then for progression upon the land." A man, by contrast, "alters his naturall posture and swimeth prone, whereas he walketh erect." Defenders of AAH take this alteration as a sign of the naturalness of natation, maintaining that human beings have a sort of diving instinct: we put our hands above our heads, they maintain, forming a sort of point that enables us to glide through the water, even if we have never been in the water before. But the most important evidence for AAH comes from what little hair the human body does have: it follows the flow lines of water.

Interestingly, the direction of body hair has, in the past, also served as a crucial bit of evidence in the controversy surrounding that other trait so often associated with the human essence: bipedality. In his 1699 anatomical study of a chimpanzee, published under the misleading title *Orang-Outang, sive Homo sylvestris*, Edward Tyson argues that the direction of the hair on the arms of the chimpanzee may serve as a sign of its proper gait: "The tendency of the Hair of all the Body was downwards; but only from the Wrists to the Elbow 'twas upwards; so that at the Elbow the Hair of the Shoulder and the Arm ran contrary to one another. Now in *Quadrupeds* the Hair in the fore-limbs have usually the same Inclination downwards, and it being here

different, it suggested an Argument to me, as if Nature did design it a *Biped*."

By convention, the great apes had long been placed in the same category as cows and dogs with respect to gait. Even Linnaeus, unable to pretend that apes' hands were feet, nonetheless held onto the conceit that they are quadru-something-or-other by deeming their feet to be hands and calling them *quadrumanes*. But the chimpanzee's hair patterns were already enough for Tyson to infer that the creature walked upright, and thus that it had exactly two feet and two hands. And uprightness, at least where no feathers are involved, has often served throughout the history of philosophy as a convenient stand-in for rationality. Tyson will go on to deny that the ape can speak, even if he cannot find anything in its physiology that would prevent it from doing so. But the floodgate is opened: in the eighteenth century, the standard assumption will be that "orang-outangs" are but degenerate men, who are only unable to speak as a result of their uncouth upbringing. Their body hair is an outward report of the poverty of their social environment.

Stand up straight. Speak clearly. Get a haircut. Near my home in Montreal, there is an epilation clinic that promises to "*faire sortir la beauté de la bête*" ("bring the beauty out of the beast.") It would not be too hyperbolic to suggest that keeping the hair in all and only the right places is, in the end, alongside language and posture, the best means we have of fixing the boundary between the animal and the human, and of keeping each our own beast hidden from sight.

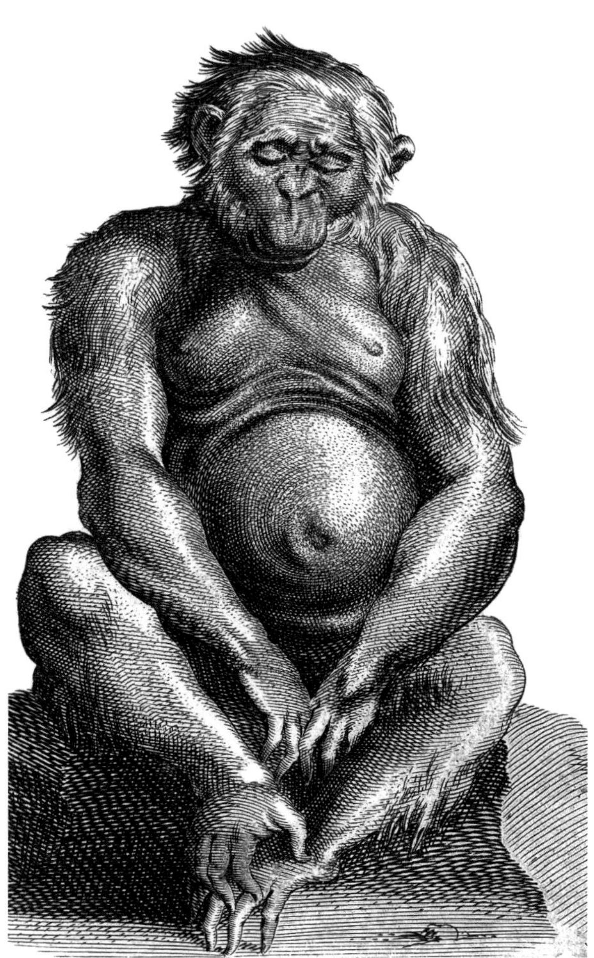

A real orangoutan, from book three of Nicolaus Tulpius's 1644 *Observationum medicarum*. Courtesy Wellcome Library.

Women (and men) with highly refined, hyper-groomed
hair have long been ubiquitous in film, television, and
advertising. For some time, seemingly effortless—but
actually highly produced—glossy, cascading curls
have been the norm for any woman appearing in the
media. Like many other "looks" for women throughout
history, this coiffure is time-consuming, and to correctly
achieve it, a crew of technicians is required. Although
I understand how artificial all this is, for me this
knowledge doesn't seem to lessen my desire to achieve
this simulacrum of falsely casual hair-perfection for
myself. As is my usual strategy, a need to paint an image
of the vexing "object" ensues, in an attempt to rid myself
of its power over me. This strategy never truly works,
but at least some paintings—such as the ones on the
following pages—are made in the meantime.

opposite: *Brunette, Curls, Purple Blouse*, 2009.
page 76: *Blond, Curls II*, 2008.
page 77: *Brunette, Curls II*, 2009.
Photos Jean Vong.

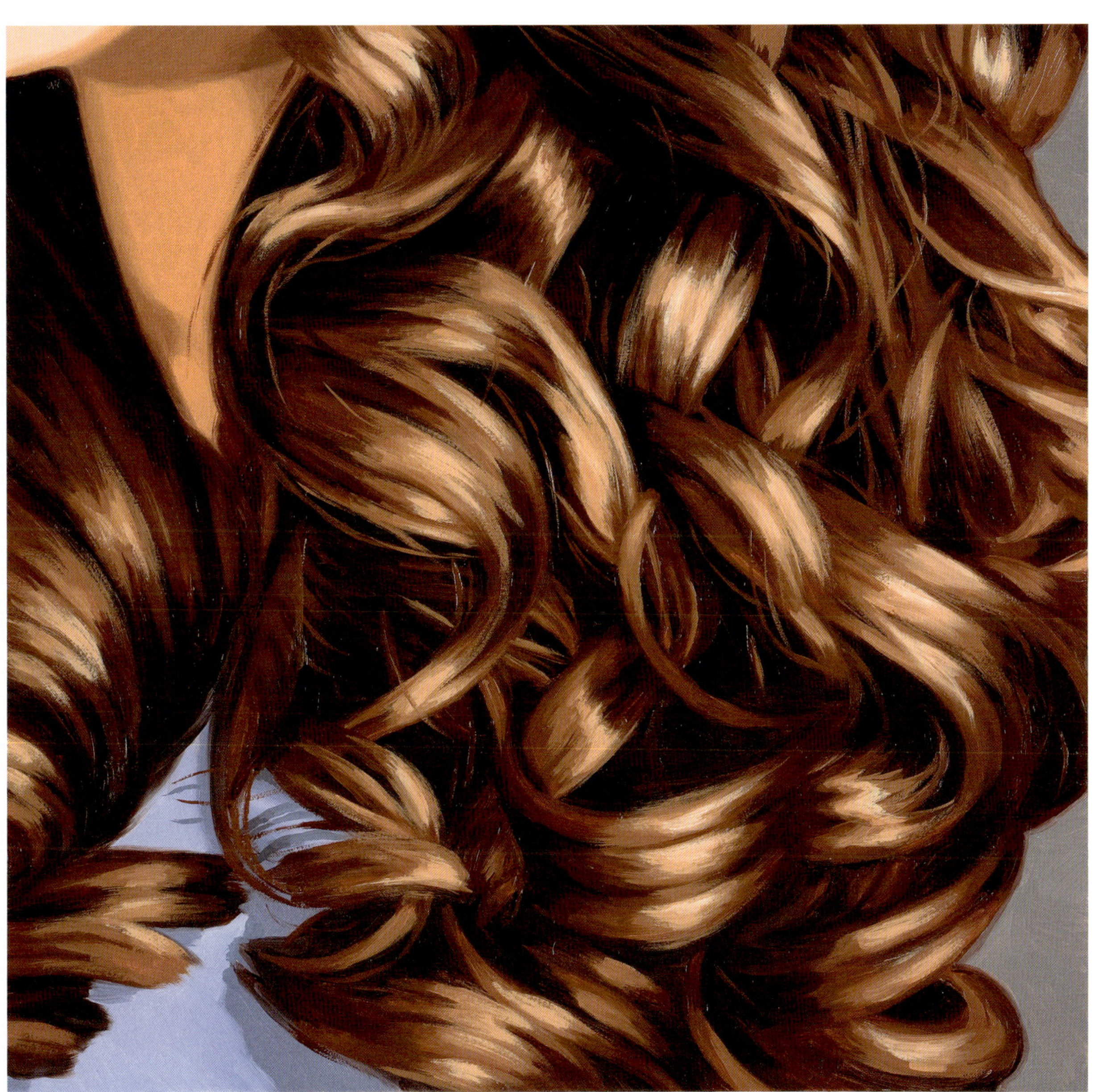

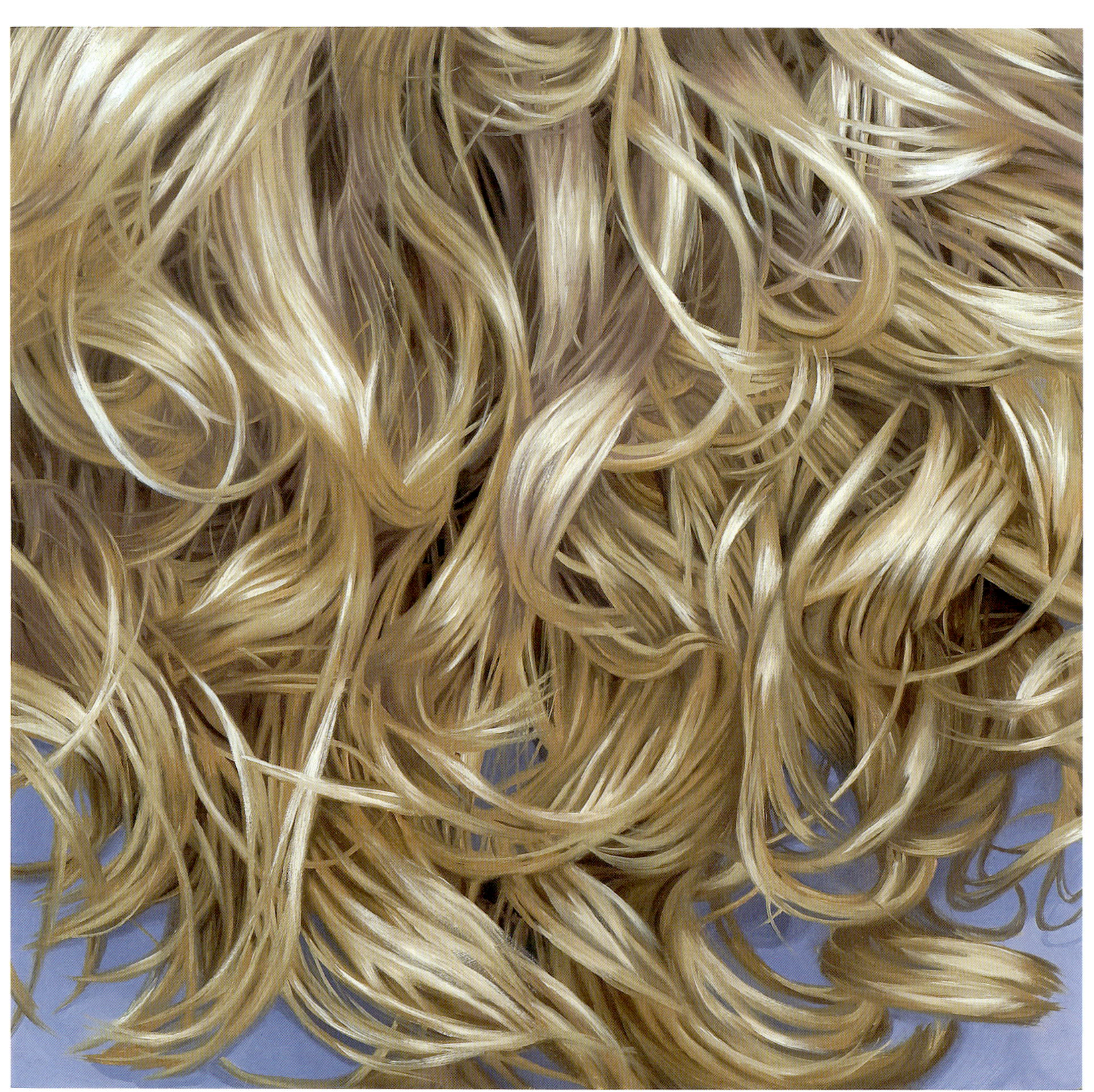

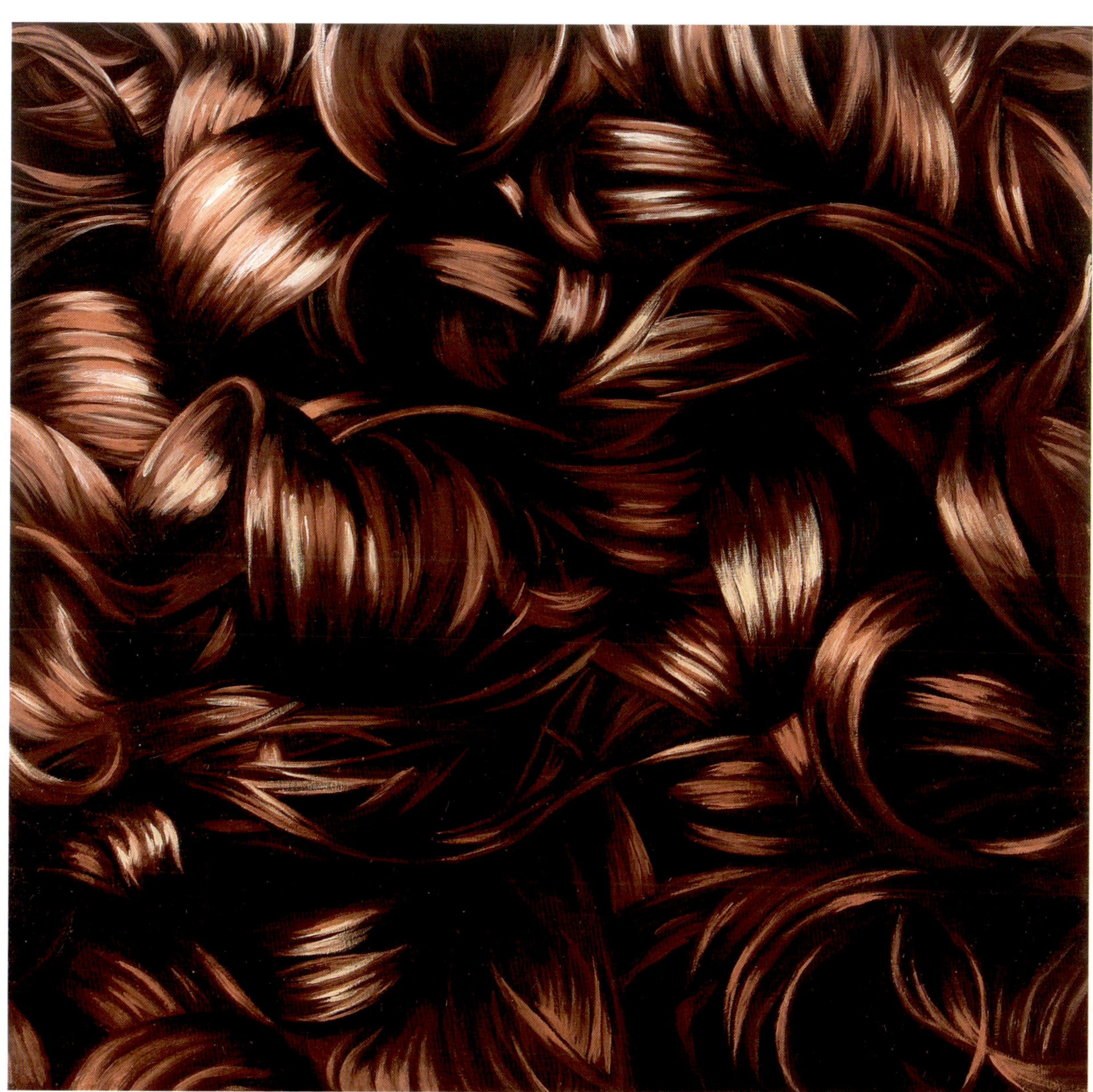

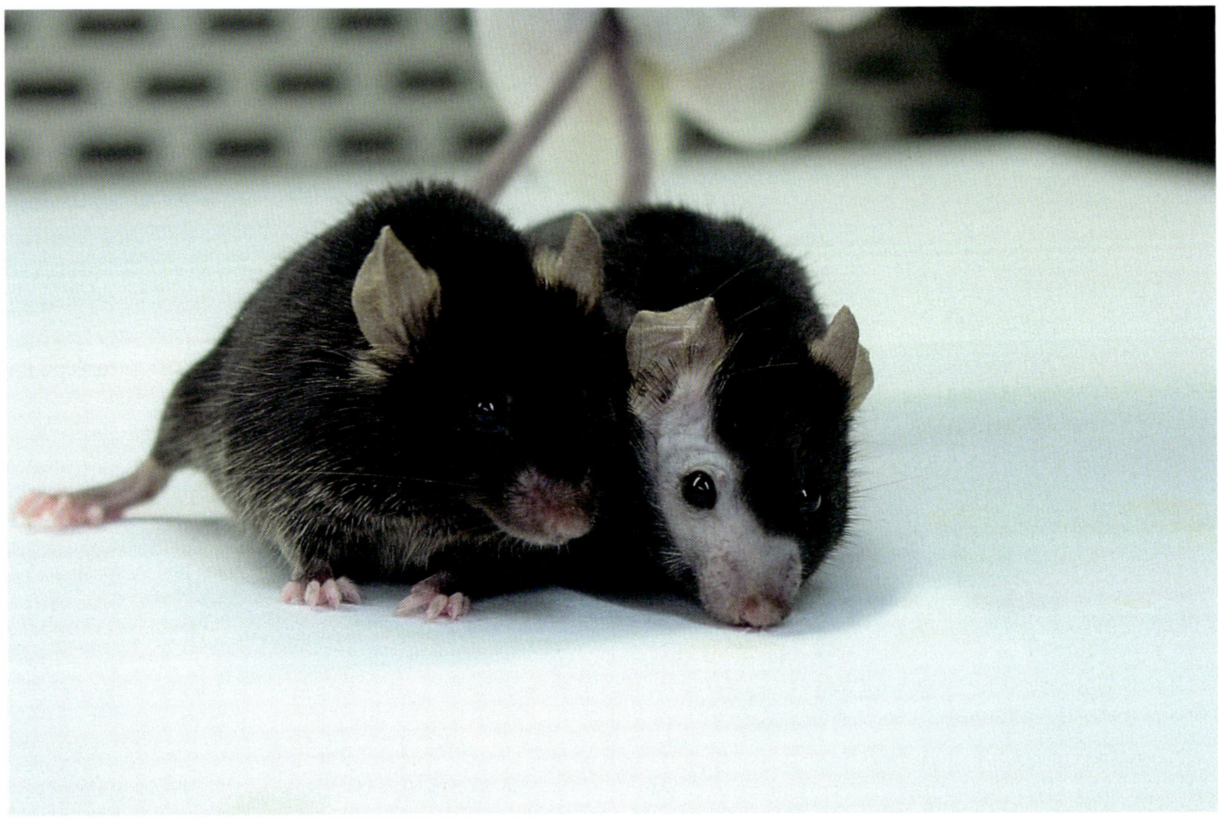

Barber mouse and a client. Courtesy Biji Kurien, Tim Gross and Hal Scofield.

OF MICE AND MANIA

LAUREL BRAITMAN

*My own brain is to me the most unaccountable
of machinery—always buzzing, humming, soaring
roaring diving, and then buried in mud. And why?
What's this passion for?*
—Virginia Woolf[1]

If you give a mouse a haircut, he might want another.
And another. And another. And it's not actually a haircut.
It's a pluck. Sometimes a nibble. When a mouse goes
to a barber, he or she loses some whiskers or some fur.
And usually it happens again and again.

Barber mice, as they are known, remove the fur or
whiskers of other mice (and somewhat less frequently,
their own). They tend to be female, but aren't always.
And they are, as far as I can tell, only to be found among
captive mouse populations, be they in laboratories or
pet owners' homes. The online message boards for
mouse-rearing humans (who raise them as pets or for
"fancy" mouse shows) are full of hair removal stories.
They post photos of mice and rats with little bald spots
on their heads, reverse mohawks, or hairless facial
patches shaped like tiny *Phantom of the Opera* masks.
Perplexed, the rodents' keepers ask questions like,
"Tache seems unable to go more than two weeks in
a cage with other mice without beginning to barber
again. ... Today I returned her to the big tank with Pu
Manchu and Mrs. Beach ... but I expect by the end of
two weeks she'll be barbering again. How to solve this
problem?"[2]

Some fanciers and breeders claim the behavior is
about displaying dominance (i.e., the barbering mouse
is boss). Others say it happens because of overcrowd-
ing or lack of stimulation: a lab mouse—even if it is
born and bred to be one—still has sensory, social, and
environmental needs that a cage, even a pleasant
one filled with exercise wheels and colorful plastic
tunnels, will have difficulty providing. What is not
debatable is that barbering is simply normal grooming
behavior gone awry. Usually mice groom by scratch-
ing themselves with their hind feet, washing their face
or fur with their front paws (using their own saliva),
and smoothing or cleaning their hair with their teeth.
Barber mice take these behaviors in a more extreme

direction by *removing* hair on others (and sometimes themselves) with their teeth. Barber mice don't usually injure the mice whose fur or whiskers they nibble or pluck. In fact, it seems that their clients may *enjoy* it—that is, they will sometimes follow the barber mouse around until she or he plucks them—even when what results is the complete loss of whiskers or an un-ironic mouse mullet.[3]

Given their extensive experience with mice in the laboratory, a few researchers have suggested that the barbering rodents might help us better understand overzealous hair removal in humans.[4] In people, repetitive hair pulling (which leaves pluckers with bald spots and sometimes even interferes with their daily life) is diagnosed as trichotillomania.[5] Not unlike mice, most human pluckers are female. The disorder affects roughly 1.5% of men and 3.5% of women in the United States,[6] though trichotillomania may be far more widespread than we think because people are often embarrassed by their bald spots and can be quite good at covering them up. Studies using mice as stand-ins for human pluckers have tried various techniques to get the mice to start barbering in the first place (that is, if they haven't started doing it themselves) and investigated the effects of antidepressants on the behavior. The fact that humans tend to pluck themselves and mice tend to pluck each other hasn't stopped the use of mouse experimental models—since both the barber mouse and her client engage in the process by choice, even when it must be somewhat painful, researchers have tended to assume, for better or for worse, that the behavior found in a single human being is simply spread between two individual mice.

In humans, the most common sites of plucking are the scalp, eyebrows, eyelashes, beard, and pubic area. People may start plucking one specific area, like eyebrows, but then, over time, switch to pulling from another region. Sufferers say that the plucking is usually preceded by some sort of tension that the pull itself releases, though it can also happen when people are relaxed or distracted (i.e., when reading a book or watching television).[7] Nevertheless, anxiety, anger, and sadness often do increase the urgency and frequency of hair pulling.[8]

There is still a good deal of confusion about how the disorder should be classified. The American Psychiatric Association's Diagnostic and Statistical Manual of Mental Disorders IV (DSM) has situated hair plucking under "Impulse-Control Disorders Not Elsewhere Classified" and counsels that this behavior should not be considered a compulsion. Unless plucking is associated with obsessive thoughts, the DSM stresses that it is also not an obsessive-compulsive disorder (since the plucking is not usually performed along a framework of rigid rules in the way that obsessive-compulsive hand-washing or lock-checking can be).

The DSM's claims notwithstanding, the behavior often does resemble a habit, an addiction, a tic, or an obsessive-compulsive disorder. More recently, researchers have begun to view it as part of a family of "body-focused repetitive behaviors," along with skin picking and nail biting."[9] Whatever its etiology, trichotillomania is in the DSM because most people don't do it. We need our hair for all sorts of reasons, some physiological, most not. Bald patches or missing eyebrows may make social situations more awkward and the time spent plucking may interfere with other things in one's life. The habit might be a symptom of anxiety or depression, but mostly it just makes the sufferer look odd and this is when it tends to be diagnosed. Some trichotillomania sufferers, particularly children, may pull hair from other people, or even pets. And it is common for people to either play with, or eat, their plucked hairs.[10]

In this, like so many of our neuroses, we are not alone. Hair pulling has been reported in six different non-human primate species, and, in addition to mice, has been observed among rats, guinea pigs, rabbits, sheep, musk oxen, dogs, and cats.[11] Just as with mice, researchers who conducted a study on feather-plucking parrots suggested that they would be a good experimental model for trichotillomania-suffering humans.[12] And like overgrooming dogs (who will sometimes lick themselves bare and oozy, a condition diagnosed as Acral Lick Dermatitis), birds have been treated with the same drugs used to treat compulsive behaviors in humans.

For captive gorillas, the most common sites for hair plucking are forearms or shins, but I have seen plucked patches wherever the apes can reach. Gorillas, unlike us, can pluck almost anywhere since they have more and thicker body hair than we do. Some gorillas, like some people, eat their hair after plucking it.

As primatologists such as Frans de Waal and Jane Goodall have observed, nonhuman animals can and do have culture, defined here as knowledge passed down from one generation to another or passed from one group to another, as in the famous case of Japanese macaques (*Macaca fuscata*) teaching one another to wash and season their yams in the ocean because the salted yams tasted better.[13] So it may be with plucking—both in people and other animals. The babies of gorillas who pluck often turn out to be pluckers

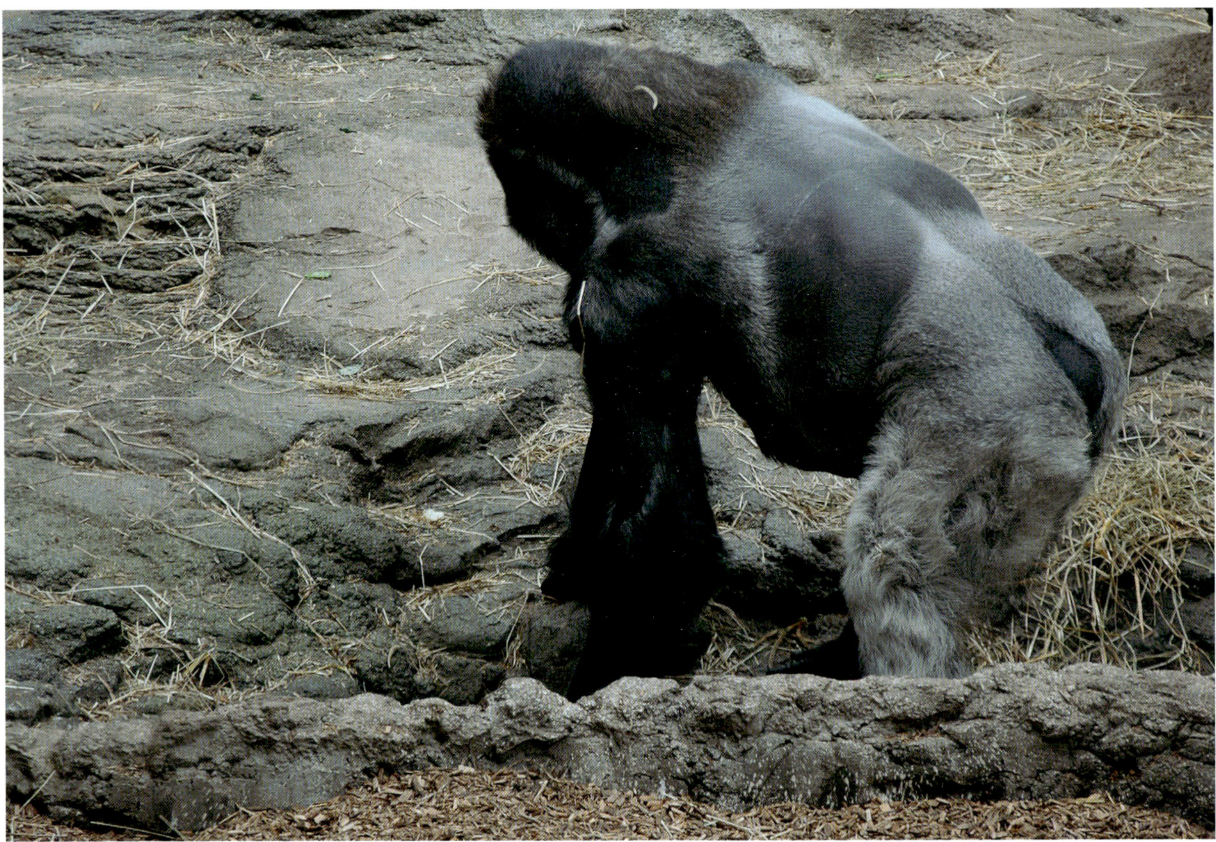

Kitombe, a male gorilla at Franklin Park Zoo in Boston, who began to pluck the hair on his head and arms more severely when he was isolated from the rest of the troop. Photo Laurel Braitman.

themselves. And troops that have never exhibited plucking sometimes start when a new plucker arrives in their midst. At the Franklin Park Zoo in Boston, none of the gorillas pulled out their hair until two young males—Little Joe and Okie—arrived in 1997 from Cleveland Metroparks Zoo. Within months, a number of the troop members in Boston were plucking.

Just as in humans, no one knows exactly why gorillas do it—except that, as it does for us, plucking may offer some sort of psychic balm or release of tension and it may be greatly influenced by one's environment.[14] There also may be a genetic component. An experiment conducted in 2002 demonstrated that mice bred without a group of key developmental genes (including the Hoxb8 gene, fundamental in the development of immune cells called microglia found in the brain) became severe self-barbers. The mutant mice didn't stop at hair trimming and whisker plucking but also used their paws to scratch bald spots and sores on their rumps. A later study, published last May in the journal *Cell*, transplanted bone marrow (containing healthy microglia cells) from a group of control mice into the population of barbers. Four weeks after the transfer, when the new microglia had made it to the mutant mouse brains, many of the barber mice (who had been using their teeth to pluck the hair on their own chests, stomachs, and sides) stopped over-grooming. In three months, their hair had grown back.[15] While no one is suggesting that human trichotillomania sufferers sign up for bone marrow transplants anytime soon, researchers are trying to understand the links between the brain's immune system and the expression of mental disorders such as trichotillomania, OCD, autism, and depression.

Like the Hox genes themselves, overgrooming behaviors may be present, in some form or another, in all vertebrates with something to pluck, lick, or pull out. While such behaviors are probably not attributable to genetics alone, a predisposition to over-grooming may exist in certain individuals, who when exposed to the right combination of stressors exhibit such behaviors. Within the avian veterinary literature,

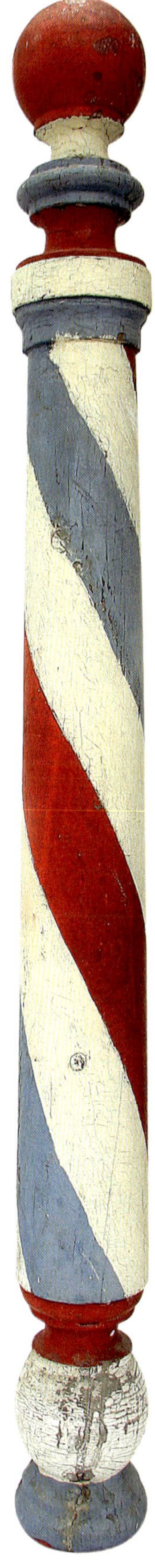

r-Picking Disorder" or
t is unrelated to a sep-
llergies—can stem
ess, or be related to
ng, attention seeking,
, and/or changes in
uld be upsetting to a

ved with parrots for
s an expert on cap-
stions from hundreds
son. She claims that
tructive behavior are
for human individu-
and helping them
rrot is healthy, ready
ntally engaged, is
ave opportunities to
However, in chronic
n useful, as have
ions.
ucked their feathers
venly) to Clomip-
sold under the brand
escribed to humans
n.[17] Another study
African greys tested
epressant, Doxepin
host parrots involved
at the Tufts Animal
documented the
c on feather picking in
ectus parrots.[18]
f this—especially
g mice, birds, cats,
whether or not these
ned light on ours.
rillas, or cockatoos
that the nonhuman
hts? Of course, we
human relationships,
ask a person what
eling doesn't mean
y may not know why
en how they feel

uarantees revelation
seek to understand
't (or won't) talk to
ne with other ani-
st another form of

anthropomorphism, but I think that is far too narrow a view. We have long looked to other animals to better understand ourselves—using them as experimental subjects, objects of philosophical inquiry, companions with whom we soothe or challenge ourselves, or as the raw material of moral lessons. Human relationships with other animals continue to center around observations and a certain amount of projection is inherent to the act of watching and interpreting what other animals are doing with their time. Our lives with other creatures are rife with instances of both good and bad projections. A human who takes Spot to the door on a rainy afternoon might see the dog pause at the threshold, nose in the air. Depending on the person, this might be understood to mean, "Spot hates going outside in the rain and so I should buy him a cute little slicker and set of rain boots so that he'll go out without a fuss."

Within the scientific community, fear of projections like this one have sometimes crippled our understanding of shared animal experience. Anthropomorphism, or the attribution of "human" characteristics to nonhuman animals or objects, has been something of a dirty word in the behavioral sciences. Such fears have long informed studies such as one I once worked on in southeast Alaska. We were observing grizzly bears and their interactions with human fishermen

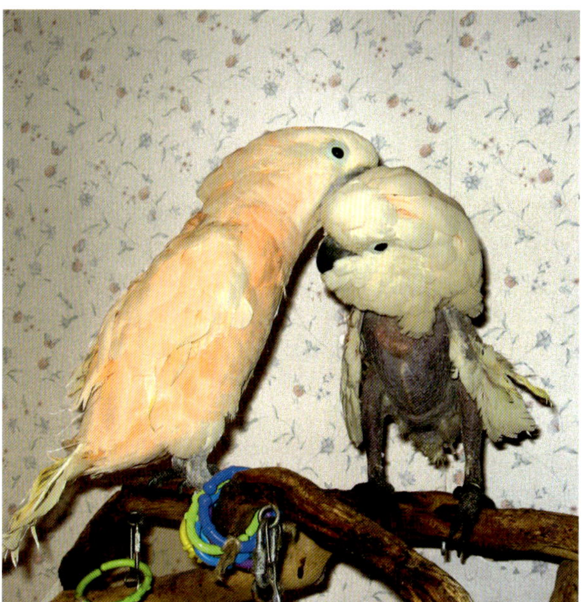

Chiquita (right) is a thirty-two-year-old female Moluccan cockatoo who arrived at Mollywood Avian Sanctuary in her present plucked condition in 2009. Eddie (left) is a nineteen-year-old male Moluccan cockatoo who has been chewing off his wing and tail feathers for ten years. He often preens Chiquita, though he does not pluck her; Chiquita, however, occasionally plucks some of Eddie's feathers. Courtesy Mollywood Avian Sanctuary.

along a salmon stream in Katmai National Park. The same bears came back summer after summer to fish, bicker, and raise their cubs and were easily recognizable by their scars, fishing styles, and personalities. And yet, as researchers, we were instructed only to use numbers to refer to the bears lest our use of human names for them might cause us to attribute human desires and thoughts to the bears as well. But outside of our official survey forms and notes, we all used names for them, like "Diver" for a bear who was fond of diving to the bottom of the river to catch his salmon. As far as I know, calling him Diver did not encourage us to assume that he was engaged in anything but bearish behavior—but that was the concern.

Thankfully, such practices have begun to change somewhat. The Stanford neuroscientist Robert Sapolsky, for example, has long used Biblical names to refer to individual baboons he studies in Kenya. Despite the holy handles, his work has not suffered and neither has that of the numerous other scientists who have more recently veered into what may have, not long ago, seemed like anthropomorphic territory. In Sapolsky's case, it may even have helped—getting to know the personalities of his individual baboons, on their own terms and his, may have encouraged him to make the leap that their stress responses approximated our own, research that has since revolutionized how we think of the affects of chronic and acute stress on the human brain.

Projecting, in and of itself, is not a problem. And if this wasn't true, animal models for mental disorders from trichotillomania to depression would simply not be as present in the scientific literature as they are. This isn't to say they aren't problematic. We cannot assume that a rat=parrot=dog=human. But if it sounds like a duck, walks like a duck, and plucks like a human—it just may be a duck we can identify with.

1 Quoted in Nigel Nicholson and Joanne Trautmann Banks, eds., *The Letters of Virginia Woolf: 1923–1935* (New York: Harcourt Brace Jovanovich, 1979), p. 140.

2 "Re: The Attempt to Save Noir from Barbering," 26 January 2010. Discussion post by Mrs. Beach available at <fancymicebreeders.com/mousefancierforum/phpBB3/viewtopic.php?f=8&t=975&start=30>. Accessed 28 November 2010.

3 F. A. Van den Broek, C. M. Omtzigt, and Anthonie. C. Beynen, "Whisker Trimming Behaviour in A2G Mice Is Not Prevented by Offering Means of Withdrawal from It," *Lab Animal Science*, no. 27 (1993), pp. 270–272.

4 Biji T. Kurien, Tim Gross, and R. Hal Scofield, "Barbering in Mice: A Model for Trichotillomania," *British Medical Journal*, no. 331 (2005), pp. 1503–1505. See also Joseph D. Garner, Sandra M. Weisker, Brett Dufour, and Joy A. Mench, "Barbering (Fur and Whisker Trimming) by Laboratory Mice as a Model of Human Trichotillomania and Obsessive-Compulsive Spectrum Disorders," in *Comparative Medicine*, vol. 54, no. 2 (April 2004), pp. 216–224.

5 The *Diagnostic and Statistical Manual of Mental Disorders IV TR* (Washington, DC: American Psychiatric Association, 2000), which is used by psychologists, psychiatrists, social workers, and others, defines trichotillomania as the "recurrent pulling out of one's own hair that results in noticeable hair loss."

6 See "Trichotillomania Learning Center FAQ," available at <trich.org/about/hair-faqs.html>, and "Pulling Hair: Trichotillomania and its Treatment in Adults, A Guide for Clinicians," a publication of the Scientific Advisory Board of the Trichotillomania Learning Center, p. 2, available for download at <www.trich.org/about/for-professionals.html>. Both accessed 28 November 2010.

7 Entry on "Trichotillomania," in *Diagnostic and Statistical Manual of Mental Disorders IV TR*, op. cit., section 312.39.

8 "Pulling Hair: Trichotillomania and its Treatment in Adults, A Guide for Clinicians," op. cit., p. 6.

9 "What is Compulsive Hair Pulling?" available at <www.trich.org/about/hair-pulling.html>. Accessed 28 November 2010.

10 "Pulling Hair: Trichotillomania and its Treatment in Adults, A Guide for Clinicians," op. cit., p. 2.

11 Viktor Reinhardt, "Hair Pulling: A Review," in *Laboratory Animals*, no. 39 (2005), pp. 361–369.

12 Patrick S. Bordnick, Bruce A. Thyer, and Branson W. Ritchie, "Feather Picking Disorder and Trichotillomania: An Avian Model of Human Psychopathology," *Journal of Behavior Therapy and Experimental Psychiatry*, vol. 25, no. 3 (September 1994), pp. 189–196. For more information on the use of drugs in the treatment of dogs, see Dora Wynchank and Michael Berk, "Fluoxetine Treatment of Acral Lick Dermatitis in Dogs: A Placebo-Controlled Randomized Double Blind Trial," in *Depression and Anxiety*, vol. 8, no 1 (1998), pp. 21–23, and Judith L. Rapaport, David H. Ryland, and Martin Kriete, "Drug Treatment of Canine Acral Lick: An Animal Model of Obsessive-Compulsive Disorder," *Archives of General Psychiatry*, vol. 49, no. 7 (1992), pp. 517–521.

13 Frans De Waal, *The Ape and the Sushi Master: Cultural Reflections by a Primatologist* (New York: Basic Books, 2001), pp. 214-216, and Bijal P. Trivedi, "'Hot Tub Monkeys' Offer Eye on Nonhuman 'Culture,'" *National Geographic News*, available at <news.nationalgeographic.com/news/2004/02/0206_040206_tvmacaques.html>. Accessed 28 November 2010.

14 Mark Lewis and Kim Soo-Jeong, "The Pathophysiology of Restricted Repetitive Behavior," *Journal of Neurodevelopmental Disorders*, vol. 1 (2009), pp. 114–132.

15 "Compulsive Behavior in Mice Cured by Bone Marrow Transplant," in *Science Daily*, available at <www.sciencedaily.com/releases/2010/05/100527122150.htm>. See also <www.unews.utah.edu/p/?r=022210-3>. Both accessed 28 November 2010.

16 Email correspondence with Phoebe Greene Linden, 5 November 2010.

17 Lynne M. Seibert, Sharon L. Crowell-Davis, G. Heather Wilson, and Branson W. Ritchie, "Placebo-Controlled Clomipramine Trial for the Treatment of Feather Picking Disorder in Cockatoos," in *Journal of the American Animal Hospital Association*, vol. 40, no. 4 (1 July 2004), pp. 261–269. See also Lynne M. Seibert, "Feather-Picking Disorder in Pet Birds," in Andrew U. Luesche, ed., *Manual of Parrot Behavior* (Oxford: Blackwell, 2008). For more on Anafranil, see <www.rxlist.com/anafranil-drug.htm>. Accessed 28 November 2010.

18 Alice Moon-Fanelli, Nicholas Dodman, and Richard O'Sullivan, "Veterinary Models of Compulsive Self-Grooming Parallels with Trichotillomania," in Dan J. Stein, Gary A. Christenson, and Eric Hollander, eds., *Trichotillomania* (Arlington, Va.: American Psychiatric Press, 1999), pp. 72–74.

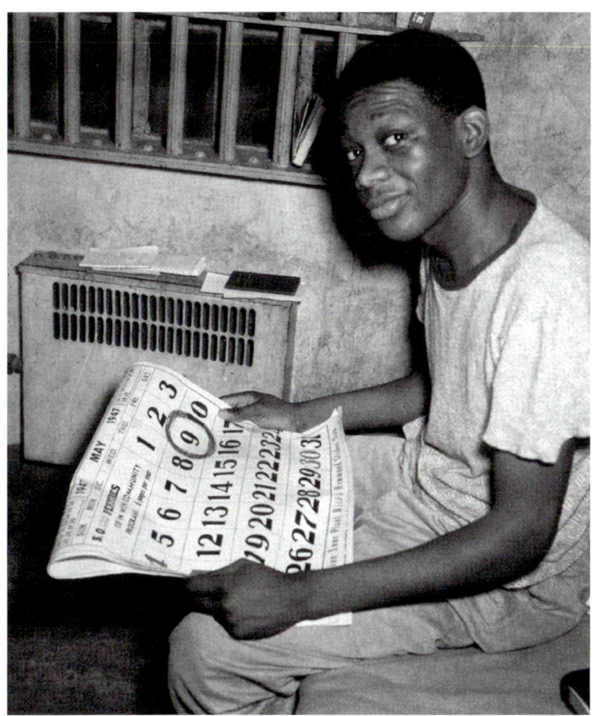

A clean-shaven Francis back in his cell after the failed electrocution of 3 May 1946.

A yet-to-be-reshaved Francis, holding a calendar with his upcoming, second execution date of 9 May 1947 encircled.

A CLOSE SHAVE WITH DEATH

MATS BIGERT

"I'm n-n-not dying" were the words coming out from under the leather hood during the electrocution of Willie Francis on 3 May 1946. "Gruesome Gertie," the electric chair used for executions throughout the Louisiana prison system, had malfunctioned and failed to produce a current strong enough for a lethal shock. The botched execution was terminated and Francis, who had been convicted of murdering a former employer, survived.

The photographs reproduced here, both of which were taken after the attempted execution, reveal one important procedure related to electrocution—being shaved. A hairless head and left calf are imperative for the effectiveness of the electric chair, the top of which is usually fitted with a tight cap containing a brass electrode and a sponge moistened with saline solution. It is through this electrode that the current—2,500 volts in the case of Francis—is introduced into the subject's body. It then travels through the trunk and exits though the electrode attached to the left leg, causing heart failure and cardiac arrest. If the body parts connected to the electrodes are not shaved properly, the resistance that the hair contributes to the circuit can prolong the time between when the current is switched on and life is switched off. It seems unlikely that hair played a role in the failure of Francis's electrocution: it is known that an inmate-barber shaved him on the day of his scheduled execution, and documents from the subsequent hearings in fact focus primarily on whether the botched attempt was due to simple mechanical failure or to the fact that the two executioners were intoxicated.

His case was finally brought before the US Supreme Court, with his lawyers claiming that Francis had already been executed, even if the procedure had failed to kill him. The argument was rejected and Francis was sent back to the electric chair a year later. On 9 May 1947, Francis was shaved for the last time.

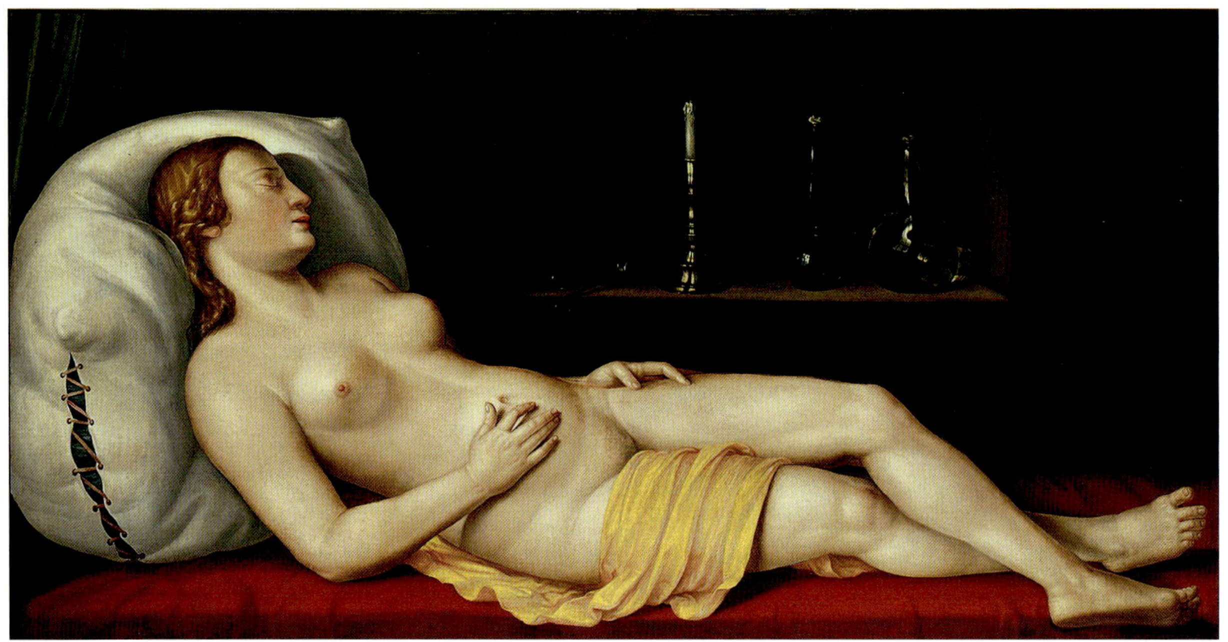

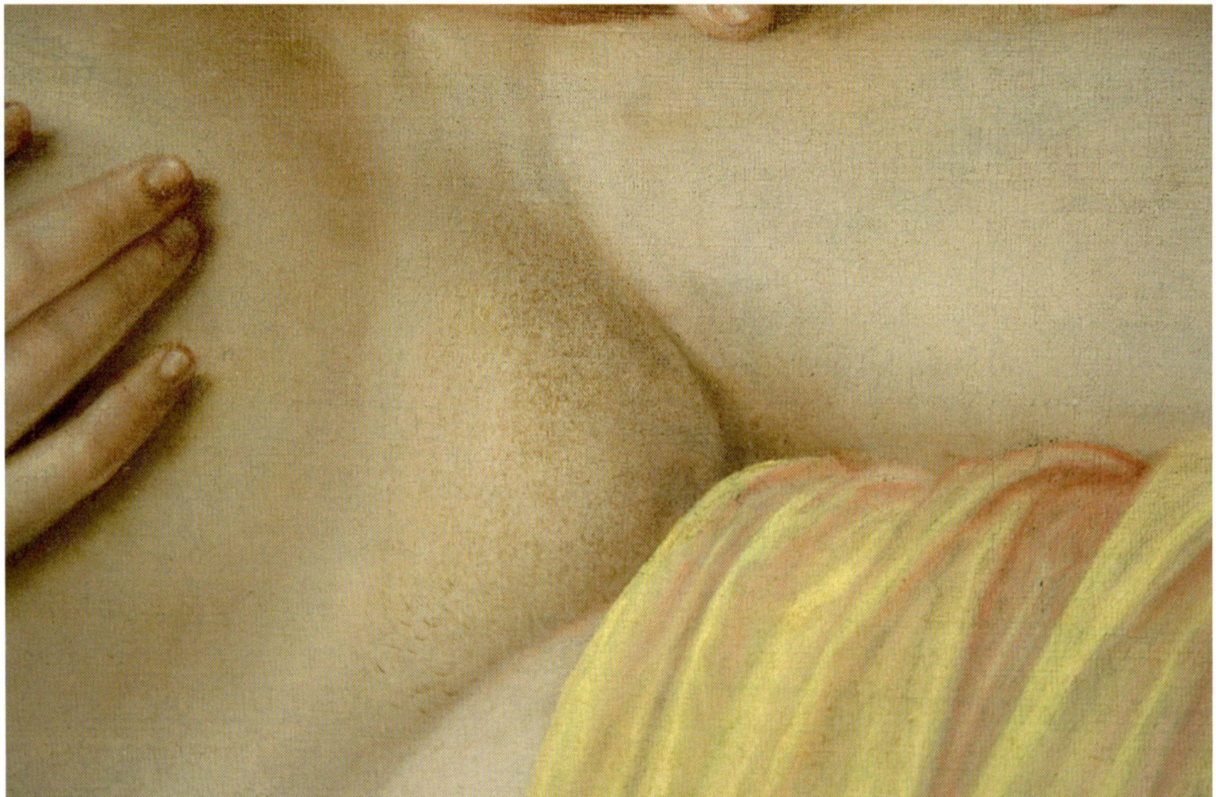

Full view of, and evidentiary detail from, Georg Pencz, *A Sleeping Woman (Vanitas)*, 1544.

ACOMOCLITICISM
BLAKE GOPNIK

Aesthetic ideals, imagined as remote and superlunary, may never be more than lowly preferences putting on airs. If only he had grasped that possibility, John Ruskin could have had a thrilling wedding night. Instead of being defeated by the sight of his bride's un-ideal pubic hair (that is one longstanding parsing of the "certain circumstances in her person" that he later said had deflated him), Ruskin could have followed many other aesthetes and artists, and simply told her he preferred her shaved.

The smooth pudenda of Western art may reflect a grounded taste for hairlessness as often as they mark aesthetic elevation. Ancient Greece, source of our later Platonisms, was an acomoclitic place. The Greeks shaved and plucked and even torched. (Although there is still scholarly debate about the precise glabrosity achieved, and its Freudian implications.)[1] Some of their later followers, rather than standing heir to a philosophical tradition, were likewise victims of a capillary fashion. "Ideal" figures such as those in Antonio Canova's hairless *Three Graces* might have gone Brazilian for "the convenience of pleasure, out of libertine curiosity and following the custom of the courtesans who modeled in Athens and Rome," as Diderot explains when he discusses hairless statuary in his 1765 *Salon*.[2] Several decades earlier, John Dryden, translating Persius's first-century *Fourth Satire*, annotates its reference to pubic depilation by citing "that effeminate Custom now used in Italy, and especially by Harlots, of smoothing their Bellies, and taking off the Hairs which grow about their Secrets. In Nero's times they were pull'd off with Pincers; but now they use a Paste, which applied to those Parts, when it is remov'd, carries away with it those Excrescencies."[3] (As late as the 1950s, Dryden's note was still being expurged from editions of his writings.) Even art history's most famously hirsute pudendum, seen in Courbet's *Origin of the World*, is less natural than it seems at first glance. Under close examination by the chief of gynecology at a major American hospital, it revealed "evidence of waxing at the bikini line."

Marcel Duchamp, though always conceived of as caring more about ideas than matter, "had an almost pathological hatred for hair," according to his first wife, and is known to have requested pubic depilation of his lovers, to match his own.[4] His art reflects his taste: the spread-legged female nude in his *Étant donnés,* the *magnum opus* of his later life, is perfectly hairless. It seems that Duchamp's smooth crotch has more to do with Burma Shave than with ancient artistic ideals and their ravishment by modern art.[5] Or rather, Duchamp may have caught on to Praxiteles and Canova as his precedents in lather.

As so often in art history, the Renaissance provides the test case for our argument. It is said that classical *ideals* were reborn among Renaissance artists, but it might be better to say that those artists caught on to classical *tastes*. In a letter published in the 1560s, the Venetian satirist Andrea Calmo wrote of a dream in which antiquity's greatest heroines, from Helen to Dido to Lucretia, gave him a depilatory powder to bestow upon his lady.[6] Granted, those heroines don't specify the powder's place of application. Upper lips, too, were kept smooth in the Renaissance.

Depilatory geography is less approximate in a shamefully neglected print from around 1540 by the German artist Peter Flötner, in which a naked woman, perhaps personifying *vanitas* or *nuda veritas*, trims her *mons veneris* with a huge pair of shears.[7] And in 1544, once again in Germany, Georg Pencz, a follower of Dürer, provides additional evidence that ought to close our case for pubic realism. Pencz's lovely painting of a sleeping nude, propped on one of the finest pillows in art, is now in the Norton Simon Museum in Pasadena. The standard take on a picture such as this would describe it as a marriage of Italian idealism and a northern commitment to the real. The ideal seems to be there in Pencz, in a hairless pudendum worthy of the Medici Venus. But his realism reveals it, once again, to be nothing more than a preferred and available option. When observed very closely—rudely closely—the model's lower belly reveals tiny flickers of black paint spaced across the pink of her skin.

Stubble.

1 See Martin Kilmer, "Genital Phobia and Depilation," *Journal of Hellenic Studies* 102 (1982), pp. 104-112.

2 "… la commodité du plaisir, la curiosité libertine, et l'usage des courtisannes qui servoient de modèles dans Athènes et dans Rome." Denis Diderot, *Salon de 1765*, in *Salons*, ed. Jean Seznec and Jean Adhémar, 4 vols. (Oxford: Clarendon Press, 1960), vol. 2, p. 210.

3 Quoted in Maurice Johnson, "Dryden's Note on Depilation," *Notes and Queries*, no. 196 (27 October 1951), p. 472.

4 Lydie Fischer Sarazin-Levassor, *Un échec matrimonial: le coeur de la mariée mis à nu par son célibataire meme* (Dijon: Presses du réel, 2004), p. 69.

5 See Michael R. Taylor, *Marcel Duchamp: Étant donnés* (Philadelphia: Philadelphia Museum of Art, 2009), p. 69.

6 The gift is "una polvere da butar via e far cazer quanti peli vu havé adosso." Andrea Calmo, *Le lettere di Messer Andrea Calmo, riprodotte sulle stampe migliori*, ed. Vittorio Rossi (Turin: Ermanno Loescher, 1888), letter 24 of book 4, p. 307. See also Lynne Lawner, *The Lives of the Courtesans* (New York: Rizzoli International, 1987), p. 28.

7 Reproduced on p. 58 of Ann Sophie Lehmann, "Op de grens: Lichaamshaar in de kunst van de Renaissance," in *De grenzen van het lichaam Innerlijk en uiterlijk in de Renaissance*, ed. Arie-Jan Gelderblom and Harald Hendrix (Amsterdam: Amsterdam University Press, 1999), pp. 47–73. This is the main text on pubic hair in Renaissance art. A better image of Flötner's print is available online in the British Museum's collections database.

ARTIST PROJECT / THE DREAMTIME
SO YOON LYM

The series of portraits reproduced on the following
pages were inspired by the artist's work as a teacher in
a New Jersey high school, where she has photographed
students for the last eight years. Focusing on the intricate patterns of hair braiding, known as corn-rows for
their resemblance to agricultural furrows, the works
(all acrylic on paper) constitute a typology that evokes
both shared ethnic and racial practices and highly
individualized expressions of personal identity.

opposite: *Jose*.
overleaf, top row: *Anthony, Jhonathan, Antonio, Hector*; bottom row:
Diosnedy, James, Quay, Mario. All images 2009–2010.

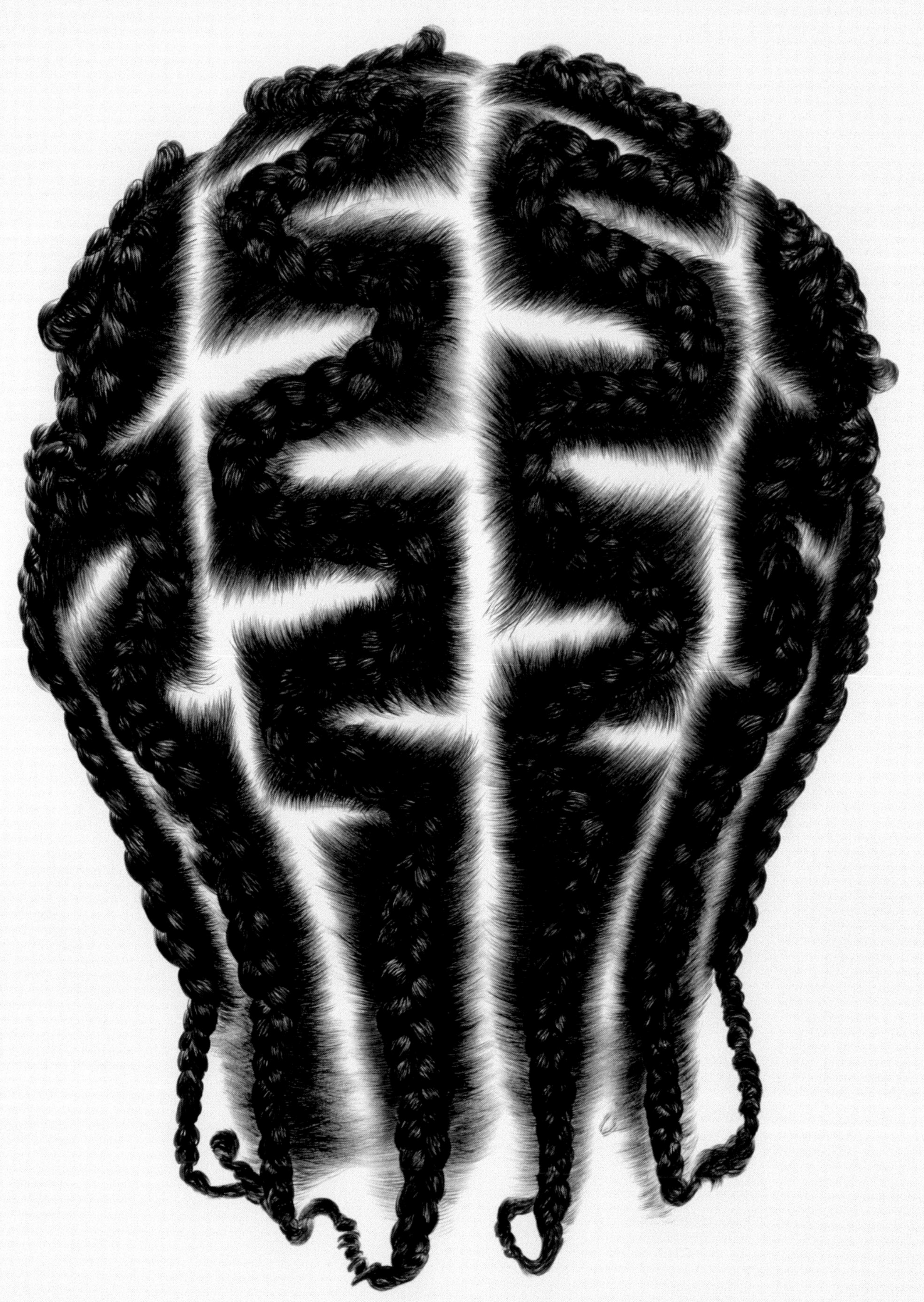

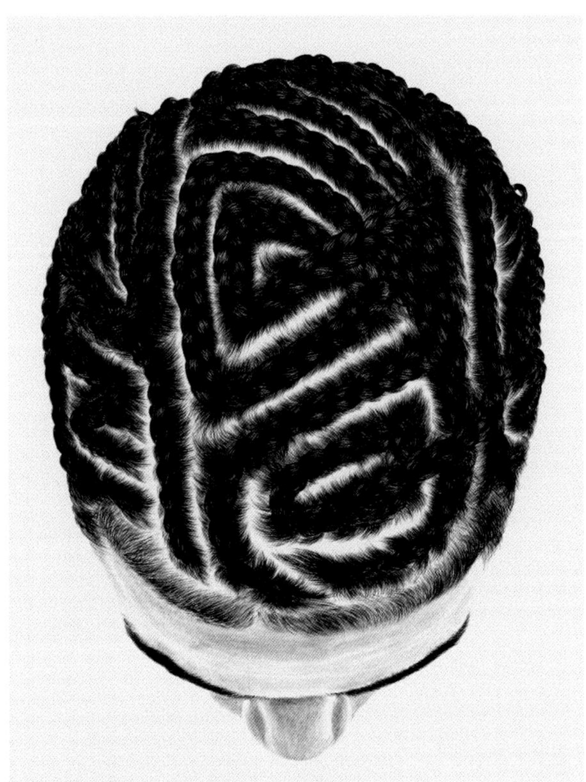
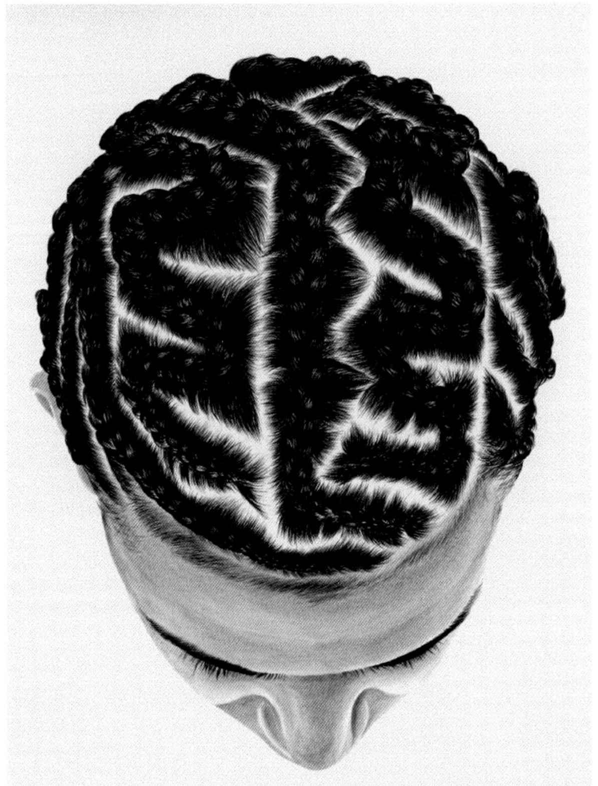
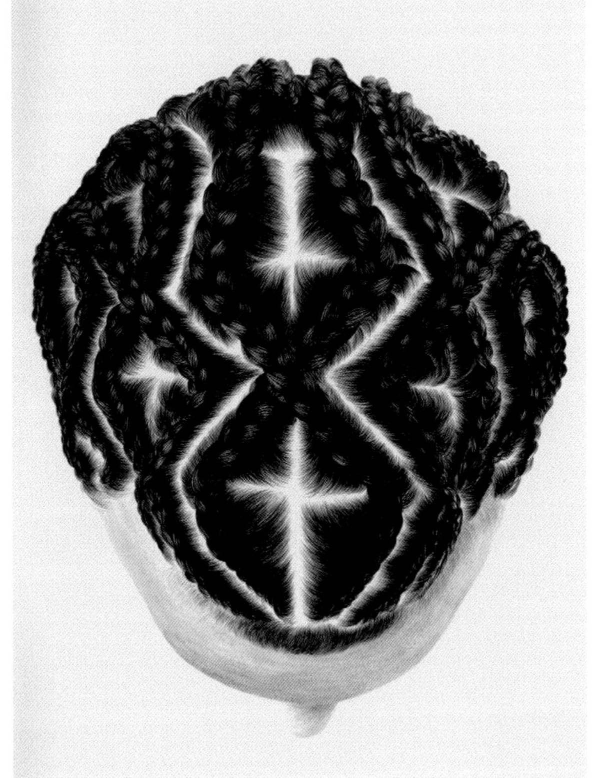
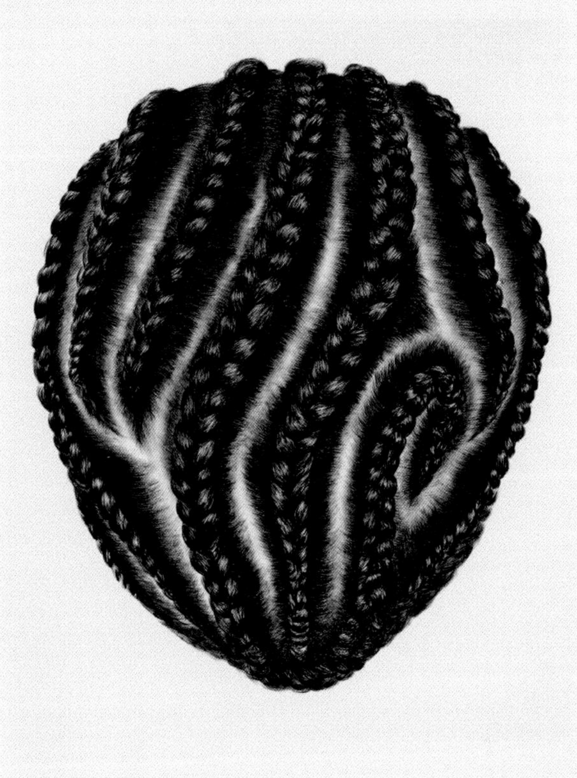

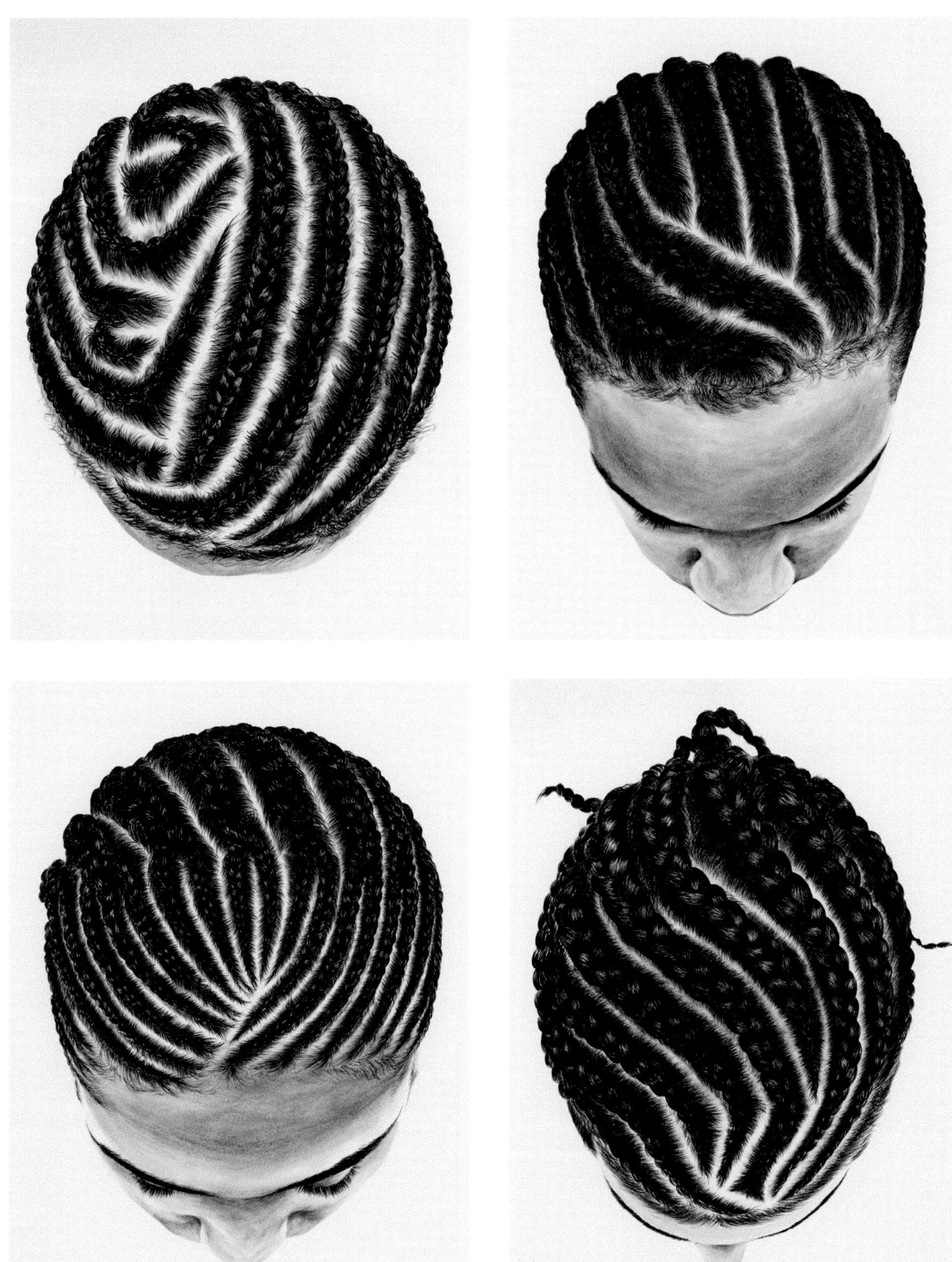

Twentieth Century-Fox Film Corporation

STUDIOS
BEVERLY HILLS, CALIFORNIA

December 14th, 1965

Dear Mia,

I am writing to you both as a friend and as an
employer.

When you came into my office Friday, after
cutting your hair, you expected me to be angry
with you. I did not show anger, because that
seemed pointless; and I didn't really feel
anger, because the potential damage was more
to you than to me or to the series or to the
studio. And that is what I am writing about
to you.

It so happens, Mia, that we are able to
accomodate the storyline to your action. But
it might very well have happened that we could
not. In that case, you would have injured all
those who depend upon this series. That is
something to consider. You have a legal contract
with us and a moral contract with all those who
work with you. And you have a conscience which
tells you both must be kept.

But going beyond that, Mia, and in keeping with
my very warm feeling for you, I must ask you
to consider carefully the effect upon your career
should people begin to feel that your impulsiveness
can impair productions. This industry, as you
know, rightly requires strict disciplines. The
strange thing is that you not only are usually
very professional but you do have a strong inner
discipline on which you can draw. If you fail
to draw upon it, as you can, naturally outer
disciplines will be imposed, and I would deeply
regret that.

I have not lost any of my feeling or regard for
you, and I hope that is of some consequence to
you. As I said in the office, you are a uniquely
beautiful girl-and-woman, and I am not thinking
of the way you look but the way you are. I wish
that you realize how gifted you have been, how
fortunate you are, how fortunate you can remain.

You have in this company and at this studio several
people who have deep and good feelings for and
about you. You know who they are. Counsel with
them, Mia, and keep faith with them.

MATTERS OF THE HEAD
EMMA MARKIEWICZ

In an account of his visit to England in 1748, the Swedish botanist Pehr Kalm reports that "Farm-servants, clodhoppers, day-labourers, Farmers, in a word, all labouring-folk go through their usual every-day duties with all Peruques on the head. Few, yea, very few, were those who only wore their own hair."[1] Accustomed as we are to a range of Hollywood images of bewigged aristocrats, we might be surprised by the widespread use of wigs in eighteenth-century England, but abundant visual and documentary evidence confirms that Kalm's observation was not anomalous. In fact, the wig was a ubiquitous part of life across the social spectrum in England in the first half of the eighteenth century until it began to fall out of fashion, and its connection to a range of social concerns provides new insight into the era's conceptions of health, hygiene, beauty, and status.

HAIR AND HEALTH

In the eighteenth century, hair was conceived of not only as an external indicator of a person's well-being but also as a part of the body that could itself be affected by ill health. In either case, hair in the medical literature was rarely seen as a separate entity and was commonly discussed in conjunction with other body parts and physical conditions. Some considered it a primary marker for the humoral condition of the head, the intellectual seat of the human body. For instance, *Aristotle's New Book of Problems, Set Forth by Question and Answer*, a 1725 volume that was part of a genre that took its form from the Greek philosopher's *Problemata*, attempted to answer the question, "Why does hair grow on the head more than any other part?" by asserting that hair is "an excrement" that grows primarily on the head because of the moistness of the brain, and is therefore likely to grow longer in women whose brains are more moist than men's.[2] The same book explains that baldness is a result of dryness, and those with curly hair, having the driest heads, are particularly susceptible to losing their hair.[3] At the end of the eighteenth century, hairdresser Alexander Stewart could still express the same understanding that hair was a humoral production: "Hair is produced from heat and moisture—too much heat dries up the substance ... too much cold, wet or dampness will prevent growth."[4] As the external, physical embodiment of the humoral fluid, the hair's appearance contained a wealth of information about an individual's health and character.

Debates about contagion and the spread of infection in published medical works frequently referenced

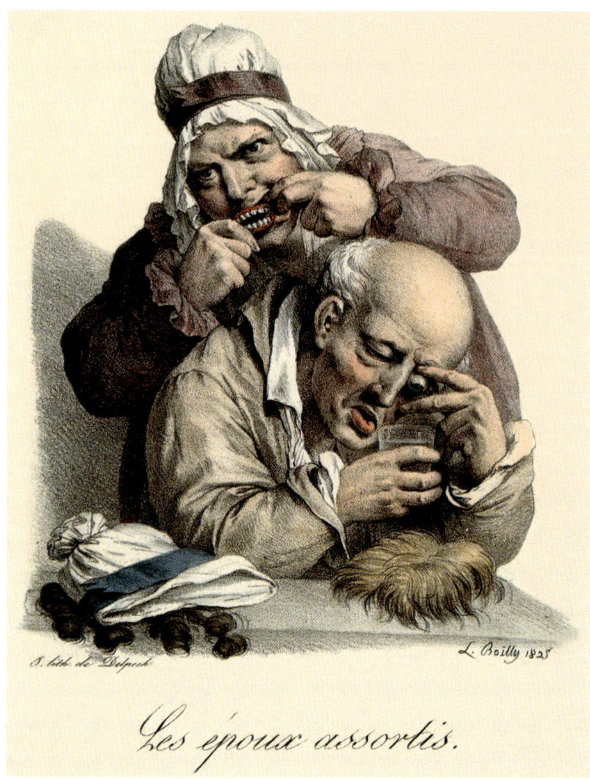

Lithograph from 1825 depicting couple as they assemble themselves using false body parts: dentures, a glass eye, and wigs. Courtesy Wellcome Library.

hair, and the hair used in wigs, as a concern. Work by seventeenth-century physicians such as Thomas Sydenham had shown that emanations from the earth—from human, animal, or inanimate matter—were contributors common to the spread of all disease. As such ideas took hold, hair, fur, and even silk or feathers came under suspicion. Derived from living creatures, these materials were believed to still contain "animal juices" and to "receive and communicate infection."[5] Unsurprisingly, during a time when the plague seemed ever-imminent, there was considerable anxiety that the hair used to make wigs may have been contagious. Stories about wigs infected with plague and smallpox travelling the country were repeated anecdotally, with one writer claiming that a wig had passed on infection from London to Plymouth. In the 1660s, Samuel Pepys voiced similar concerns, writing: "Up, and put on my ... new periwigg, bought a good while since, but darst not wear it because the plague was in Westminster when I bought it."[6] This anxiety was found not only among physicians, hair merchants, and those living in busy, dirty cities, but also in the trade laws of the day. A Parliamentary bill from the late 1740s specifically referred to human hair as "more especially liable to retain infection, and may be brought from Places infected into other countries, and from thence imported into his Majesty's Dominions."[7] It was recommended that hair being brought into Britain should be subject to an order of quarantine. Likewise John Brooks, a wigmaker who also traded hair, submitted a memo to the Treasury in 1756 stating that he would like to inspect "humane and brute hair" being brought into the country for "plague and any other Contagious Distemper whatever."[8]

Some physicians questioned the reality of the problem, however, wondering why doctors' medical wigs were not responsible for a great deal more spreading of infection than was believed to be the case. Richard Mead (1673–1754), a physician who made a study of transmissible disease, was also less inclined to blame the doctor's wig for the spread of infection, setting out a theory that certain "plague keepers" could only transmit the disease if the air was bad at the same time.[9]

HAIR AND DOMESTIC CLEANLINESS

From the late seventeenth century, the enduring view that divine intervention and internal imbalance were primary causes of disease was beginning to be overtaken by the belief that nature and infected airborne vapors were responsible. Smelling good was one way to control the external environment in your immediate vicinity, even if the good smell served to mask something dirty beneath. Judging from the numerous powders, pomatums, soaps, oils, and combs on the market, keeping the hair clean and pleasant-smelling was certainly a primary concern, and these cosmetics were commonly advertised by hairdressers and perfumers to fulfill that cleansing function. Hairdressers resorted to creative means when marketing their own powders, emphasizing how other cheaper products made with chalk or marble dust could clog up the hair and hinder respiration, having the potential to cause bodily imbalances leading to headaches and other maladies.

It was not uncommon for hairdressers to publish their own manuals on caring for and dressing the hair; in addition to containing useful information for clients on the importance of keeping their hair clean, these often also served the additional function of advertising products and services. Rather than undergoing a continuous process of shedding and renewal, as we understand today, hair was believed to accrue strength, which it sustained into maturity. As a result, hairdressers argued it was worth investing in the health of one's hair from a young age.

The complicated and expensive hairstyles sported by many fashionable women during the eighteenth century meant that they were unlikely to comb their hair, sometimes leaving it untouched for months, leading one commentator to wonder if they had to apply mercury in order to keep away lice, the scourge of all social classes in this period. Already in his 1665 book *Micrographia*, Robert Hooke (1635–1703) had made some detailed and radical observations about lice using microscopic lenses. Hooke's examination had shown that a louse was able to cling on to an individual hair using its claws, which enabled it to feed from blood vessels in the scalp.[10] A century before Hooke, when a humoral understanding of the body was unchallenged, nits had been seen as an unavoidable aspect of daily life, with hygienists attributing them to the excess of humors and uncontrolled substances emanating from within the body. Hooke's work with the microscope was groundbreaking as it showed that lice "proceed from [the eggs of] parents of their own kind, and not (as formerly was supposed) from certain juices or humours of human bodies."[11] This new understanding suggested that individuals could affect whether they were infested with lice, and that they could control the presence of nits by maintaining certain levels of external cleanliness in their hair, skin, and clothes. Lice, of course, were perfectly visible without the use of a microscope, much to the disgust of Pepys, who in 1667 describes refusing a wig from his barber, as it was "full of nits."[12]

Pepys's disgust highlights the changing attitudes to cleanliness apparent towards the end of the seventeenth century. By the time he was writing, the notion that dirt could be controlled externally meant that it had become a social concept, not just an internal, corporeal one. Thus the greater importance given to the appearance of cleanliness, and the demonization of dirt as a threat to decency and order.[13] This shift in attitude is one prominent factor in the increasing popularity of wigs, as the need to crop or shave the head in order to accommodate a wig helped reduce the likelihood of lice infestation, not to mention the fact that hairdressers could clean false hair with greater ease and regularity.

HAIR AND BEAUTY

Contemporary hairdressing manuals stated that for hair to be considered healthy, and therefore beautiful, it should be strong and thick enough to grow long and fall down the head and shoulders. The frequent examples of concoctions detailed in both published and domestic recipe books to grow hair long, to thicken it, and to cure baldness would seem to suggest that this aesthetic was upheld in everyday life.

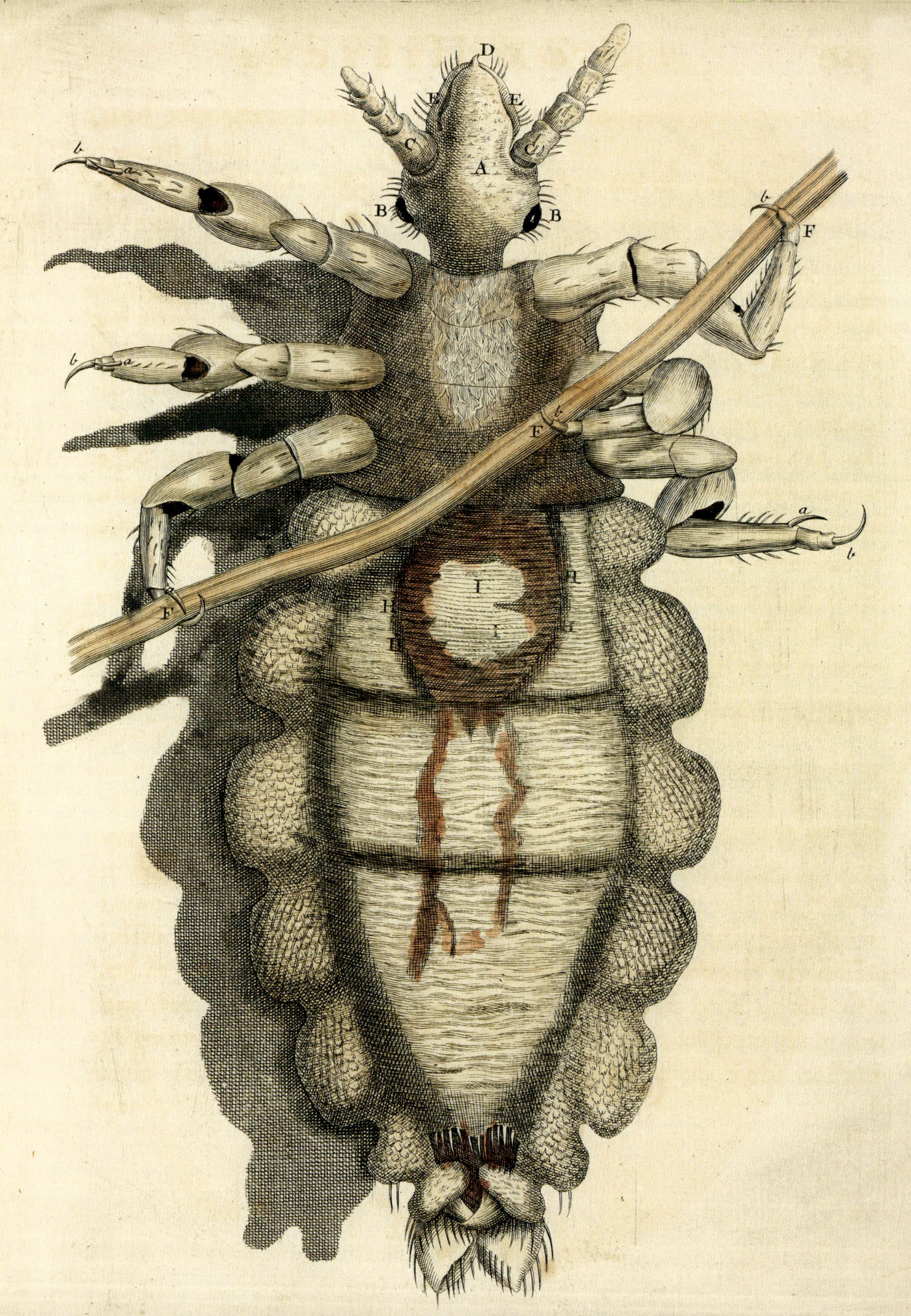
D
E
E
C
C
A
B
B
F
F
F
a
b
b
a
b
a
b
H
I
I
I
H
K
K

For many people in the eighteenth century, a look of youthful beauty was only available for a fleeting period. City dwelling, harsh physical work, a propensity for diseases which left permanent physical scarring, and simply growing old all made the image of attractive health nearly impossible for the majority of working people to maintain. But this was not simply an issue of class. People situated in higher socio-economic groups, such as the independently wealthy or those in professions affording a more genteel lifestyle, were also at risk of disfiguring diseases, to say nothing of obesity and problems with joints and movement that resulted from overindulging in life's pleasures.

Then, as now, it was common to employ artifice to maintain socially mandated aesthetic standards. Using cosmetics to hide imperfections on the face, powders and dyes to disguise the graying color of hair, and stays and underclothes to change the silhouette were all popular tactics. Of course, wig wearing was a crucial part of this regimen. In one case, a man was observed to tie a thick tape in the back of his wig, pulling it tightly to compress his temples and face, thus giving himself an instant face-lift and reducing the appearance of sagging skin.[14] A similar technique that involved tying a ribbon under the arms and hiding it with a wig could correct bad posture in children.[15] In addition to projecting an image of a healthy body, wigs could disguise an unhealthy one, covering scars from medical procedures, hiding disfigurements, or camouflaging physiological defects requiring medical intervention such as a hearing aid.[16] Wigs could likewise be used to protect a wound after an operation, or to prevent an abscess or ulcer from making contact with the air.[17]

THE BUSINESS OF HAIR

With all the various uses for wigs, the matter of procuring hair was absolutely vital for wigmakers—human hair, of course, being the most desirable and expensive. In 1730 a new tax was proposed on the use of "brute hair, such as cow and calves' tails, mohair, horse, goat and camel's hair,"[18] which was being passed off as human hair and bringing wigmakers into disrepute. The same document also proposes a second tax upon the use of French hair, as this was thought to be the most common type of human hair used at this time and was obviously perceived to threaten the domestic market.

opposite: John Carwitham, "Louse Clinging to a Human Hair," 1736. The engraving, after an illustration from Robert Hooke's 1665 *Micrographia*, appears in Eleazar Albin's 1736 book *A Natural History of Spiders, and Other Curious Insects*. Courtesy Science and Society Picture Library.

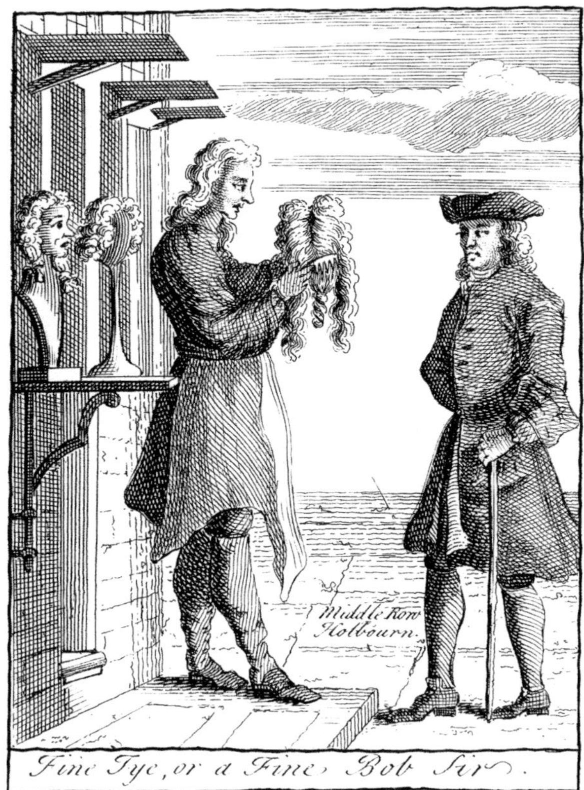

A London wigmaker entices a client with his wares in Middle Row, Holborn. Date unknown. Courtesy Wellcome Library.

Customs records detail the "hair humane" that was brought into London ports, imported in the largest quantities from Flanders, France, Holland, and Spain (to the value of approximately £33,500 in today's money from Spain alone in one month during 1726).[19] It arrived in lesser quantities from Italy, Portugal, and "East Country," along with horsehair from Russia. There is no record of hair being exported in its raw form, but quantities of perukes were sent to Germany, Russia, Turkey, and England's overseas territories (Barbados, Jamaica, New England, New York, Carolina, and the West Indies).[20]

Judging from period documents, trading in hair had the potential to be the most lucrative area of the business. In 1756, John Brooks of Holborn recorded sales of parcels of French hair worth £90,000 (roughly £6.5 million today).[21] Harvey Spragge, recorded as a "Hair and Silk Merchant," was said to have died leaving a fortune of £30,000 in 1733.[22] At the other end of the social spectrum were itinerant chapmen, who often sold human hair, particularly in the late seventeenth and early eighteenth centuries at the height of the wig's popularity. Urban hair merchants are known to have employed dealers to purchase hair from around the country and it is possible that some exploited the chapmen's communication links. Another way to procure hair was to make it come to you, as can be seen from advertisements placed by barbers and wig-makers with offers such as this: "If any man or woman hath good hair to sell, let them repair to George Gray Barber and Perriwig maker over against the Greyhound Tavern in Blackfriars, London; there they shall have at least as much ready money as anybody else will give."[23]

Hair merchants were also often responsible for the sorting, dyeing, and curling of the hair prior to selling it to barbers and wigmakers. This breadth of work meant that these businessmen were often the largest employers in the entire industry and maintained the widest trading networks. The larger merchants also employed "pickers" to sort through the hair and select the best quality hanks, arranging them into colors and winding them onto rollers for curling. For the latter work, many merchants maintained connections with bakers who would bake it for a nominal fee. Of course, some merchants were wholesalers who sold the hair untreated, suggesting a certain crossover in which wigmakers, barbers, and merchants could all be responsible for undertaking the preparation of the raw material. This would have made it harder for the customer to be sure of the quality or provenance of the product, making the wigmaker's relationship with the customer of paramount importance to economic survival.

A clean, well-appointed shop would have been particularly vital for those engaged in the hair trade in order to attract customers, particularly in an urban environment where competition was high. House visits were also common, with practitioners splitting their time according to demand—typically spending three days in the shop and three days making visits. In many larger towns, different occupations had their own districts, which the wealthy and fashion-conscious would have been familiar with and visited to acquire various goods. In London, wigmakers often set up shop in the West End and the Strand, situated in what was already an important area for textiles and clothing, as well as an entertainment district where members of high society would gather to see and be seen.

The idea generally accepted by fashion historians is that the wig came to England from France in the second half of the seventeenth century through the court of Charles II. Large, bell-bottomed wigs, which were hugely expensive items using enormous amounts of hair, were certainly popular at court and among the upper classes, setting off as they did a rich, grand, and dignified silhouette when paired with embroidered coats, long waistcoats, and lace ruffles. But despite these lofty origins, an extensive network of hair practitioners did develop to supply the lower classes with cheaper forms of wigs. In 1727, Daniel Defoe asserted that there were thirty thousand barbers and wigmakers in London alone.[24] This figure is almost certainly a deliberate exaggeration—especially considering that estimates in the 1750s suggest the total population of the city was approximately eighty-seven thousand—but the exaggeration does dramatize how this strange prosthetic, which Defoe observes was "little known" in England fifty years before, came to be a ubiquitous fixture on the heads of both aristocrats and commoners.

1 Pehr Kalm, *Kalm's Account Of His Visit to England On His Way To America in 1748* (London: Macmillan and Co.,1892), p. 52.

2 Aristotle (pseud.), *Aristotle's New Book of Problems, Set Forth by Question and Answer*, sixth edition (London: John Marshall, 1725), p. 32.

3 Ibid., p. 80.

4 Alexander Stewart, *The Natural Production of Hair or its Growth and Decay, Being a Great and Correct Assistance to its Duration* (London: self-published, 1795), p. 5.

5 Richard Mead, *A Short Discourse Concerning Pestilential Contagion, and the Methods to be Used to Prevent It* (London: no publisher given, 1720), p. 77.

6 Latham, ed., *The Diary of Samuel Pepys* (London: Bell and Hyman, 1985), p. 520.

7 British Parliamentary Papers, 1747, vol. 9, "A Bill to Oblige Ships more Effectually to Perform their Quarentine; and for the better Preventing the Plague being brought from Foreign Parts into Great Britain, or Ireland, or the Isles of Guernsey, Jersey, Alderney, Sark, or Man."

8 The National Archives, T1/370/27, "The Humble Memorial of John Brooks Peruke Maker and Dealer in Hair and Corn" (1756).

9 Richard Mead, *Some Remarks on Three Treatises of the Plague* (London: Sam Buckley & Ralph Smith, 1721), p. 20.

10 Hooke, *Micrographia* (London: The Royal Society, 1665), p. 64.

11 Ibid.

12 Latham (ed.), *Diary of Samuel Pepys*, op. cit., p. 746.

13 Georges Vigarello, *Concepts of Cleanliness* (Cambridge: Cambridge University Press, 1988) p. 79.

14 William Rowley, *The Rational Practice of Physic* (London: no publisher given, 1793), p. 358.

15 Andry De Bois-Regard, *Orthopaedia: or the Art of Correcting and Preventing Deformities in Children* (London: A. Millar, 1743), p. 95.

16 Lorenz Heister, *A General System of Surgery in 3 Parts* (London: no publisher given, 1743), p. 435.

17 Richard Wiseman, *Eight Chirurgical Treatises, on these Following Heads* (London: Benjamin Tooke and John Meredith, 1705), p. 433; Pierre Dionis, *A Course of Chircugical Operations Demonstrated in the Royal Gardens at Paris* (London: Jacob Tonson, 1719), p. 458; Charles Gabriel Le Clerc, *The Compleat Surgeon: or the Whole Art of Surgery Explained*, fifth edition (London: R. Bonwicke et al., 1714), p. 36.

18 Anonymous, *Some Considerations on the Present State of the Hair Trade* (London: no publisher given, 1730)

19 This figure was derived using the National Archives currency converter, avilable at <www.nationalarchives.gov.uk/currency>.

20 The National Archives, CUST 3/ 28A, 1726.

21 The National Archives, T1/370/27, 1756.

22 *St. James Evening Post* (London), no. 2752, (16 January 1733).

23 *Intelligencer Published for the Satisfaction and Information of the People* (London), no. 13 (February 1665).

24 Daniel Defoe, *The Compleat English Tradesman*, vol. 2 (London: Charles Rivington, 1727), p. 167.

ON THE DIRECTIONALITY OF HAIR

SPYROS PAPAPETROS

Often invoked as a metaphor of irrationality and confusion, hair in the nineteenth century was also employed as an instrument of scientific precision. From criminological investigations to anthropological inquiries, hair was presented both as material evidence and as a methodological pattern, whose minute accuracy helped scientists direct their research towards the *root* of a problem. More than texture, form, and color, however, the most revealing quality of hair in scientific research of that period was its *direction*—hair's geometric capacity not only to occupy but to delineate space, including the realms of knowledge.

In his 1856 lecture on adornment, the nineteenth-century architect Gottfried Semper used hair and hair ornaments as indicies of spatial direction (*Richtung*).[1] Hair could be used to form "pendants" (such as the long beards and heavy hair braids of the ancient Assyrians which hang down symmetrically), or "rings" (such as the annular coiffures of ancient Greek women forming a circular corona around the head). But Semper also distinguished a third type of adornment, for which the architect coined the term "directional ornament" (*Richtungsschmuck*). These adornments accentuated the orientation of a subject in movement, and included the warrior's fluttering garments, headgear, or windblown hair, as well as the decorated mane of military horses (such as those depicted in the famous reliefs from Nimrud, which Semper would have seen at the British Museum while he was in exile in London).

Drawing from the etymology of the Greek *kosmos*, which meant world, order, adornment, as well as direction and discipline, Semper bestowed each of his three ornamental categories with a cosmic attribute. While pendants and rings were respectively linked to macrocosmic equilibrium and microcosmic proportion, directional ornaments were representative of a world in flux—a dynamic universe whose human and animal bodies were gradually substituted by the eidetic signs of their accessories. Thread-like appendages such as hair augmented the subject's corporeal volume while reducing its presence into a transient vector. While singular in direction, the same vector pointed to a manifold transformation. The fabric of the world was constantly changing, and cultural theorists and evolutionists alike attempted to decipher that new texture by dissecting its mobile edges—the appendages of clothing accessories and hair extensions.

One of the many readers of Semper's essay on adornment was the evolutionist and amateur anthropologist Emil Selenka, who was a colleague of Karl Semper, a professor of morphology and a nephew of the architect. Both scientists had spent a considerable amount of time traveling in the German colonies of Southeast Asia, collecting natural specimens and writing travel memoirs describing their encounters with indigenous cultures in which they analyze the dress, adornment, and hair arrangements of native tribes, including the texture, color, and peculiar mode of hair style.[2]

Selenka eventually wrote a treatise titled *The Adornment of People*, in which he applied Semper's categories of rings, pendants, and directional ornaments to adornments from non-Western cultures.[3] The anthropologist would illustrate Semper's "pendants," for example, by depicting the long hair braids of Indian fakirs, and directional ornaments by the feather headgears of North American Apaches. However, the most telling of these studies on the "rudimentary" forms of ornamentation were contained in the scientist's evolutionist studies.

Selenka was the leading scientific authority in the study of "ape-humans" (*Menschenapfen*) or *pithikanthropoi*—the various species of primates that preceded *Homo sapiens*—as well as the main editor of a multivolume series of comparative studies on the evolution of these species, including the structure of their teeth, bone, and hair. One of these illustrated volumes, titled "On the directionality of hair in ape-embryos" (*Affenembryonen*), contains a detailed examination of growth patterns in the fur of young apes within the main three primate species.[4]

Scientists had already established that hair grew in geometric patterns that have multiple centers located differently in each species. Evolutionists then followed the direction of hair strands from their origin to their end point in the extremities, tail, face, belly, and anus. The decisive evidence that would lead scientists to a conclusion was in the devilish minutiae down to the level of follicles.

Hair threads move either in a radial or spiral direction from a center; they form "streams," as indicated in diagrams such as the one presented here, by a series of arrows. These demarcated hair flows emulate electromagnetic currents which can converge or diverge with one another and create ornamental patterns such as crosses and rhomboids. The numerous drawings of young apes traversed by myriad directional arrows transformed the animal body into a force field: a quasi-cosmological diagram expanding inside the

outline of a baby monkey. Extremities such as toes and
fingers provided an outlet for that proliferating energy
to be channeled back into the world. Here, hair is still a
form of adornment in Semper's "cosmic" sense: these
minute arrows not only extended the animal body into
the world, but also reinscribed all cosmic forces *directly*
on the surface of the animal epidermis. Adornment
was no longer an external pendant or a ring, but an
entire field of directions by means of which the body
realigned itself with the forces that enveloped it.

From the linear symmetry of man in Semper's
physiomorphology of culture to the directional flow
of ape hair in the diagrams of turn-of-the-century
evolutionists, a cosmological shift had occurred: ornamentation had not disappeared, but retreated to its
origins by folding back into the skin—the living vestige
of a primal surface.

1 Gottfried Semper, "Über die formelle Gesetzmässigkeit des Schmuckes und
dessen Bedeutung als Kunstsymbol," in *Monatsschrift des wissenschaftlichen
Vereins in Zürich*, no. 1 (1856), pp. 101–130.
2 Emil and Lenore Selenka, *Sonnige Welten: Ostasiatische Reise-Skizzen*
(Wiesbaden: Kreidel, 1896) and Carl Semper, *Die Palau-Inseln im Stillen Ocean:
Reiseerlebnisse* (Leipzig: Brockhaus, 1873).
3 Emil Selenka, *Der Schmuck des Menschen* (Berlin: VITA Deutsches Verlag-
shaus, 1900).
4 Gustav Schwalbe, "Über die Richtung der Haare bei den Affenembryonen
nebst allgemeneinen Erörterungen über die Ursachen der Haarrichtungen,"
(based on findings by Emil Selenka), in Emil Selenka, ed., *Menschenaffen*, vol. 5
(Wiesbaden: Kreidel, 1911).

opposite: The directionality of hair in embryo of *Macacus cynomolgus*.
Elements from plate 4, volume 5 of *Menschenaffen*, 1911, edited by Emil
Selenka.

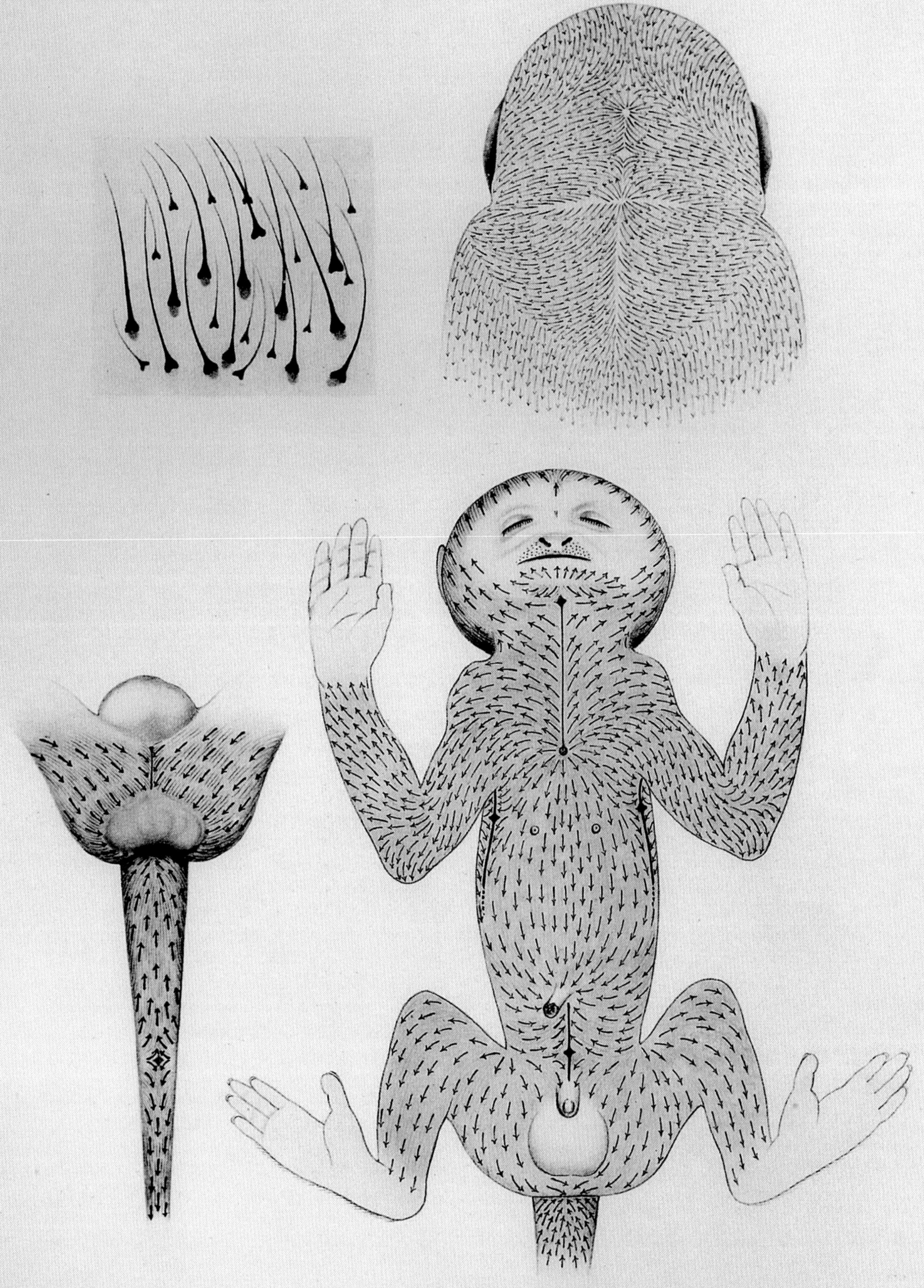

BARBERS AND BARBARIANS

JORIAN POLIS SCHUTZ

In Argentina, you see boys wearing their hair long and wild. For this, shampoo must be foregone for weeks and haircuts for months so that maximum unctuousness may be achieved. The savage impulse must withstand the perennial opposition of forces for shortness—for there is always a national mythology of hair to grow out of and into. The goal is to achieve a look that embodies a descriptor that a century ago would have conveyed deep derision, but which today in Argentina means "awesome" or "perfect": *bárbaro*.

Argentina is one of the places in the world where the hairdo of European "civilization" has most earnestly (and anxiously) been worn. This is a country that spent more than a century looking back over its shoulder, longing to restore the umbilical connection to a Europe that largely peopled its shores, while horrified to face its own uncivilized interior—the vast Pampan expanse. Hair became one site for this national psychodrama between civilization and barbarism.

I.

Much of this story has played out under the auspices of a particular shiny bald dome—that of Domingo Faustino Sarmiento, whose 1845 classic *Facundo: Civilización y Barbarie* sets the scene. Equal parts history, biography, sociology, polemic, and prose-poem, *Facundo* paints a mythical world divided between the enlightened forces for Argentine unification and the animalistic energies of local *caudillos* (military strongmen who dominated Argentinian politics at this time) such as Juan Facundo Quiroga (1788–1835), whose appetites, temper, preternatural animal sense, and, of course, bestial appearance are given full play in Sarmiento's text:

> *Facundo is a type of primitive barbarism. He recognized no form of subjection. His rage was that of a wild beast. The locks of his crisp black hair, which fell in meshes over his brow and eyes, resembled the snakes of Medusa's head.*[1]

Facundo, portrayed by Sarmiento as illiterate, would perhaps have been gratified by such a grand mythico-literary treatment. But whatever he actually was, this "tiger of the plains" became the original *gaucho malo*, or outlaw, a libidinous giant on the frontiers of the nation, his face "sunk in a forest of hair."[2]

Sarmiento later became president of Argentina,

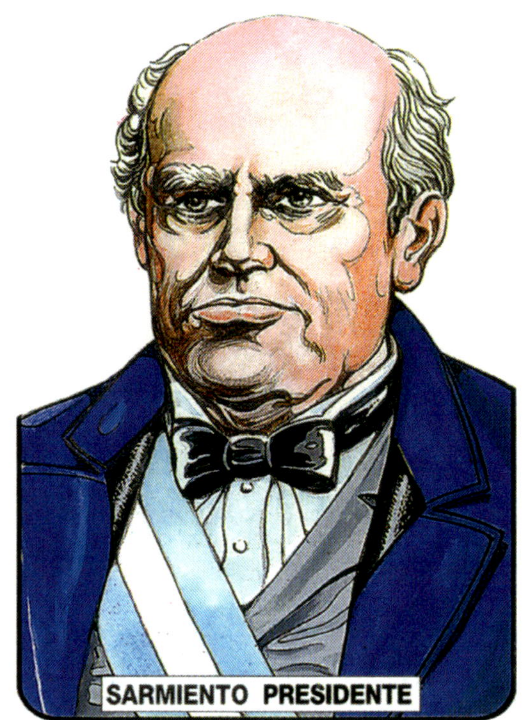

Sticker produced for the annual Argentine celebration of Sarmiento on 11 September.

ushering in an age of modernization, immigration, and manifest-destiny-style military advance that ultimately made the frontier and all of its fast-disappearing barbaric inhabitants into phantasmal objects of national nostalgia. This he did in part by invoking on his mythical spectrum the opposite of the animalized interior of his own nation. Already, in his influential book of travel essays, published as *Viajes* (1851), Sarmiento had praised above all the jewel in the crown of the dynamic North American scene—the "Brahmanic race of the United States," the inhabitants of New England. These Northerners disciplined their new populations, inculcating them with their own ethic in schools, in books, in elections, and in all their other institutions. From this dissemination of the spirit of enterprise came the great achievements of civilization and colonization—the railroads, banks, societies, and so on.

Sarmiento called New England his "fatherland of thought" and proposed to establish a corresponding elite in Buenos Aires. Fueled by European immigration and progressive education, this cadre of what we might call "barbers of barbarianism" was to be charged with the responsibility of replacing the cattle ranch with the factory, the wild horseman with the disciplined rower, and all communication inefficiencies with the lightning-quick telegraph. A new nation, to be called the United

States of the Río de la Plata, was to be forged from a united Argentina and Uruguay. "Our Pampa makes us indolent," Sarmiento proclaimed, "and the easy feeding of our shepherds keeps us stuck in incompetence."[3] Sarmiento declared war on the zeitgeist of his nation, and it was hard not to listen to him—even long after his death. "Sarmiento the dreamer continues dreaming us," wrote Jorge Luis Borges in poetic tribute.

II.

In the hands of José Hernández, perhaps Argentina's second most important stylist, the *gaucho* that Sarmiento hated became a man to admire, and the wildness of frontier hair became a model for a quintessentially Argentine head. *El Gaucho Martín Fierro* (1872) is the story of a conscripted country man who, after fighting for years in an endless war of national expansion, decides to desert, discovers that he has lost his family, becomes a vagrant criminal, and ultimately seeks refuge among the indigenous *bárbaros* that he had originally been ordered to fight. All along, honest verse pours out of the mouth of this used-and-abused figure, "like sheep, one after the other," offering rustic wisdom that redeems the world of the marginalized animal-man.

Hernández's anti-Sarmientanism dates back at least to his first published work from 1863, *Vida del Chacho* (The Life of Chacho), a vitriolic polemico-hagiography that directly inverted the *Facundo* scheme by converting one of the *caudillo*'s allies into a true man of the people and Sarmiento into a cold-hearted assassin, indeed a *bárbaro* himself, a sort of South American Sweeney Todd:

> *General Peñaloza has been beheaded. The man ennobled for his unquenchable patriotism, his strength for the sanctity of his cause, the Argentine Viriathus, in front of whose prestige the conquering forces were smashed, has just been riddled with stab-wounds on his own bed, his throat slit and his head presented as proof of an assassin's job well done, to the barbarian Sarmiento.*[4]

Hernández was sent into exile by Sarmiento in 1870, just as Sarmiento had been sent into exile by the dictator and cattle baron Juan Manuel de Rosas thirty years before. And, like Sarmiento with *Facundo*, exile gave Hernández the impetus to conceive on the mythical plane and the tranquility to conjure the Pampan figure that would become the most beloved in Argentine literature. Within the world of *Martín Fierro*, the forces for civilization and progress are revealed to be the very same that destroy the *gaucho*'s idyllic rooted life and turn him into a drunken killer. The expansion of the nation is shown to be a truer definition of barbarism, and the much-maligned long hair of the *gaucho* is valorized as a symbol countering the dehumanizing forces that press on him from above.

III.

Long hair was not outlawed during Argentina's military Proceso dictatorship (1976–1983), but it might as well have been. Authorities were waging a constant war against *juventud sospechosa* ("suspicious youth")—hippies, *rockeros*, communists, left-wing Peronists, and homosexuals, all of whom were associated with the wild-hair look. The *bárbaro* had moved into (or emerged from) the city—and was now dubbed *terrorista*.

This was the age of the dawning of *rock nacional*, and messy heads were all over the scene. Government agents began breaking up concerts with tear-gas and detaining the *rockeros* that resisted. Albums with subversive content were censored or banned, and many artists were forced into exile. *Rockeros* met clandestinely in urban parks on weekends to exchange underground albums and publications. These were the years when thousands of people, mostly young, were disappearing without trial or trace. Wearing long hair was no joke, and no innocuous fact. It was an act of resistance that could only be made viable *en masse*.

This story has roots in two rather different "coiffure classics" from the previous dictatorship (1966–1973), when the state was first confronting homegrown rock music. In 1968, the RCA-backed band La Joven Guardía released "El Extraño con el Pelo Largo" (The Stranger with Long Hair):

> *Wandering through the streets,*
> *watching the people go by,*
> *the stranger with long hair*
> *goes, without worrying why*

The song became one of the biggest hits of the nascent Argentine rock scene and was converted into a highly successful film of the same name, as well as a somewhat less successful follow-up album, which was co-promoted with Coca-Cola. Here was a great song with a Beatles-derived sound and a vague, acceptable kind of rock hair.

And then there was Pedro y Pablo's social protest anthem, "Marcha de la Bronca" (March of Fury, 1970), which suffered a rather different fate:

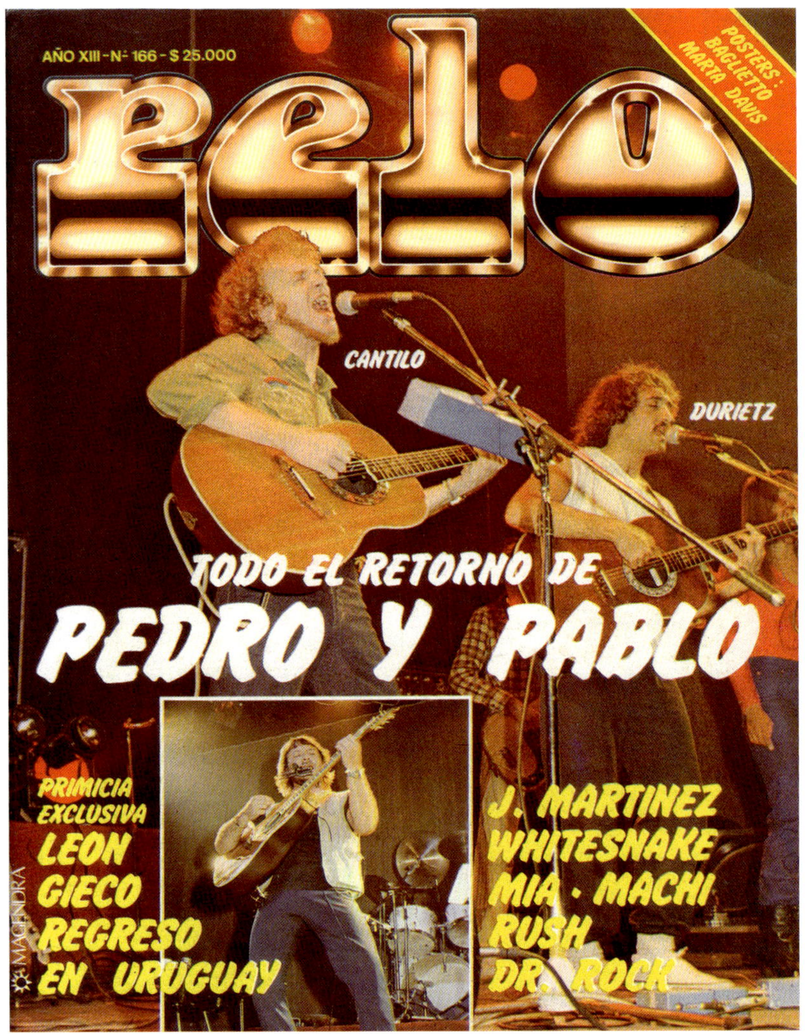

Cover of the influential music magazine *Pelo* (Hair), featuring the return of Pedro y Pablo, 1982.

Fury when they want me
to cut my hair without reason;
it's better to have free hair
than freedom with hair gel

The song came to be identified so closely with the passions of the young generation that its sequel, "La Leyenda del Retorno" (The Legend of the Return), was snuffed out by government censors and didn't appear for another eight years. Later, under the far more severe Proceso dictatorship, Pedro y Pablo's frontman Jorge Cantilo was forced into exile; when he was allowed to return in 1981—after General Videla had been replaced with the less hard-line Roberto Viola—it was only on the condition that he abandon the Pedro y Pablo name and never again sing "Marcha de la Bronca." Here was

a style that was more than a look, that brought heads together with pumping fists, and that retained its potency even a decade later.[5]

IV.

The Argentine soccer team was not always known for their long hair, as they have been in recent decades. Uniformly clean-cut players lit up the field in the 1950s, dazzling the competition at the Cópa America in 1957. But the cream of this crop was snapped up by Italian recruiters, and the remaining team was dealt devastating defeats in the 1958 World Cup—a watershed in the history of Argentine sports. The subsequent reforms of the Asociación del Fútbol Argentino along European lines nicely complemented the post-Perón political ethos of foreign-directed modernization but in fact backfired.

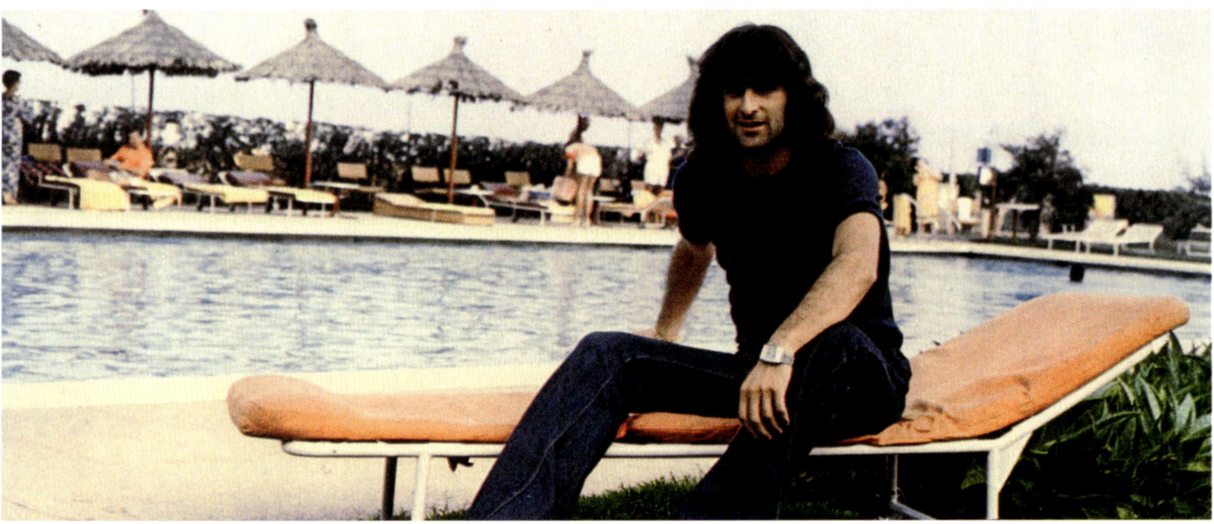

Mario Kempes, Argentinian striker who scored two goals in the 1978 World Cup final against the Netherlands. Here, he and his hair are seen relaxing by the pool.

The Argentine national team—professional, administrated, technocratic—floundered throughout the 1960s.

It was only with the rise of César Luis Menotti's club Huracán in the early 1970s that an inspiring new style of Argentine play—and, indeed, footballer—was forged, and thus it was that on the eve of the 1978 World Cup, which Argentina was to host, the military regime found itself in the uncomfortable position of depending on a ragtag team of longhairs to deliver them a new sense of national pride. Menotti, a left-wing Peronist who himself wore shoulder-length hair, had been appointed to coach the national team by the administration of Isabel Perón in 1974. The team was traveling in Poland in 1976 when the military coup occurred, and upon its return Menotti offered his resignation. But the military junta needed this victory, and they dared not take the helm from Menotti—or the role of mascot from the mop-headed cartoon character *Gauchito*. Plus, in the wake of the heavy suppression of *rock nacional*, the authorities were glad to have Argentine youth focusing on a somewhat more controllable arena for passionate behavior and wild hair. The uncomfortable alliance resulted in a World Cup victory, one shared by long- and short-haired forces alike.[6]

It was the 1978 team that solidified the Argentine "look" on the world stage, with Kempes, Luque, Bertoni, Houseman, the goalie Filliol, and Menotti himself sporting variations on the wild look. Strange, then, that hidden in their midst was something of a budding renegade—Daniel "Kaiser" Passarella, their captain, who would return to coach the country's team for the 1998 World Cup. Now shorn and serious, Passarella famously mandated that his players cut their hair to be part of the team. Apparently this provision led to a high-profile break with one of Argentina's most popular players, Gabriel Batistuta ("Batigol") who was consequently absent from the tournament. Interviewed later on television, Passarella responded to criticisms with a dose of professional rhetoric:

> *I answer with my work. I wake up early every morning. I go to work. This is my product, and I've come to work. … It's not a military attitude, because it's not that I like hair to be short. Not at all. But there are studies about this. They've done analyses of the players … the number of times they touch their hair when they have it long and when they have it short. I think it's a discourtesy. Long hair is dangerous.*[7]

1 Domingo Faustino Sarmiento, *Facundo, or Civilization and Barbarism* [1845] (New York: Penguin Books, 1998), trans. Mary Mann, p. 83.

2 Ibid., p. 74. Translation modified. Mann renders the phrase as "half-buried in this mass of hair," but Sarmiento's original text uses the word *bosque* (forest). Facundo was nicknamed "the tiger of the plains."

3 Domingo Faustino Sarmiento, *Argirópolis* [1850] (Buenos Aires: H. Consejo Deliberante, 1961), pp. 82, 84. My translation.

4 José Hernández, *Vida del Chacho* [1863] (Buenos Aires: Del Dock, 2005), pp. 15–16. My translation.

5 It seems especially fitting that all these socio-cultural convulsions were documented in *Pelo* (Hair), the leading music magazine of the era, founded in 1970.

6 René Houseman would later remark on the team's political ignorance: "I didn't know what was going on in the country. Today I know, and it disgusts me. I gave my hand to Videla; today I'd prefer to cut it off."

7 Daniel Hadad, interview with Daniel Passarella, 2009, available at <www.youtube.com/watch?v=8kWErRklkZc>. Accessed 2 December 2010.

SPLIT HAIRS

CHRISTOPHER TURNER

Alfie West (1901–1985) holds the world record for splitting hairs. On eight occasions, he succeeded in splitting a human hair seventeen times into eighteen parts. In so doing, he performed the impossible, the act which pedants and quibblers are accused of always hopelessly trying.

His *Leaf of the Lime Tree*, a hair divided into radial veins, is inscribed on the verso: "World Record No 6. One human hair split into 18 parts, televised by Japan 1980." His clinical incisions are as precise and magical as writing on a grain of rice, but the red annotation is rendered in clumsy and clunky capitals, like those that might be inscribed on a paranoid's sign warning of doomsday. Some of West's descriptions have fetishistic frisson: "One 14 inch split in the brunette's hair. Sealed forever, 1970."

West, an enthusiastic amateur cyclist who represented Britain in the 1929 World Championship Road Race in Switzerland, lived in London his entire life. He learned his hair-splitting technique during World War I, when he worked in a factory making aircraft parts and was taught how to grind the edge of a razor to make it as sharp as possible. He later worked as a furniture restorer and gave his hair pieces, which he framed and hung in a self-made museum in his apartment, whimsical names like *The Crossed Swords*, *A Boa Constrictor*, *A Monarch's Crown*, and *Epping Forest*.

In 1981, the writer David Coxhead discovered West's work and, after the artist's death four years later, he acquired twenty of his drawings. (In a local newsletter an obituarist confessed: "Some of us, if we are strictly honest, did sometimes cross the street with a wave, a little hurriedly, to avoid another long tale of how many follicle-ended hairs had been split into how many more almost invisible antennae.") In 1997, Coxhead's partner, the artist Susan Hiller, exhibited West's hair art in an installation at the Hunterian Museum of the Royal College of Surgeons—the ideal home for this outsider artist, a surgeon of sorts.

All works reproduced here courtesy the collection of David Coxhead. All titles and verso text given in captions preserve West's original spelling and grammar.

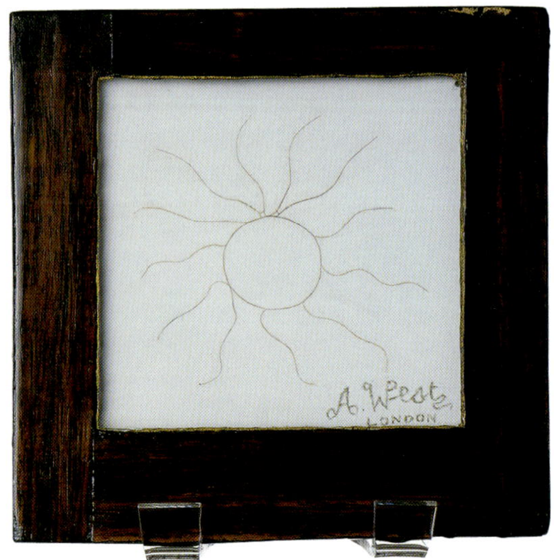

Alfie West, *The Sun in Splender with Eyes on the Universe*, 1971. Verso text reads: "Showing the Sun's two diamond 'eyes' plus 12 split parts, 1971. Guinness Book of Records since 1976 unchallenged."

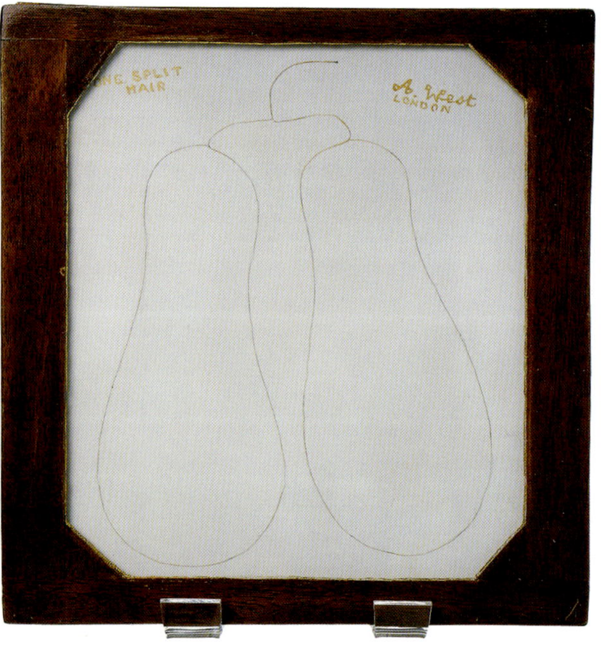

Alfie West, *The Giant Twin Pears are Just One Split Hair*, 1970. Verso text reads: "One 14 inch split in the brunette's hair. Sealed forever, 1970."

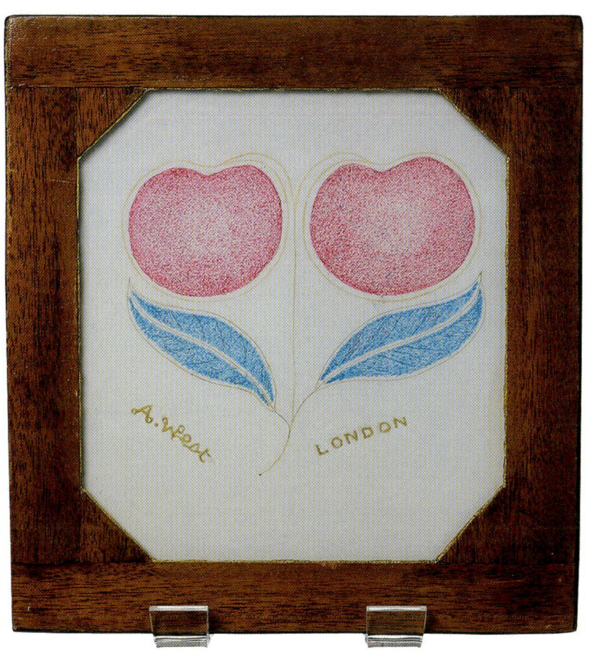

Alfie West, *Twin Roses with My Hair <u>One</u> Hair*, no date. Verso text reads: "13 split parts and 2 ace of diamonds."

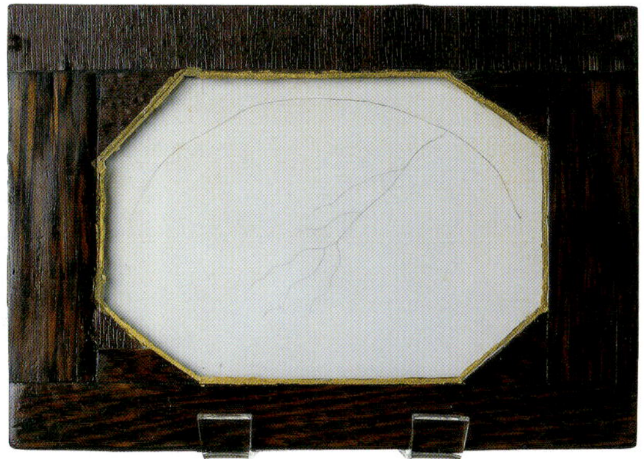

Alfie West, *Fork Lightning Flashes from a Hair*, 1960. Verso text reads: "One shaving has been cut down this hair, and no more. But that fine shaving has been split into five parts to make fork lightning. 1960. Guinness Book of Records. Unchallenged since 1976."

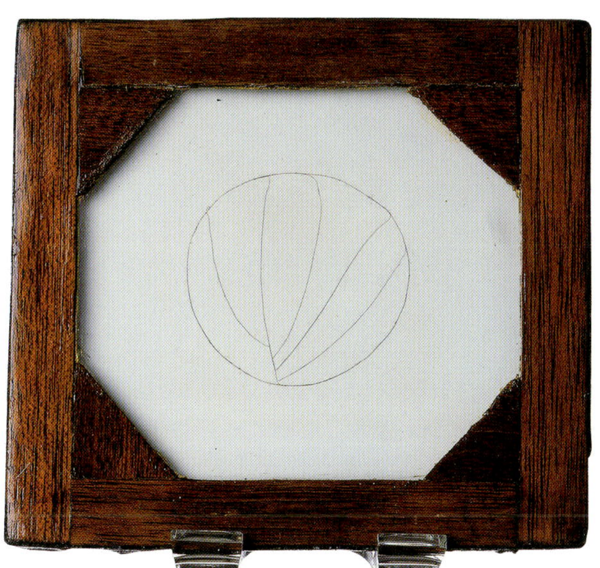

Alfie West, *The England Football*, 1965. Verso text reads: "7 split parts are seen with this hair 1965."

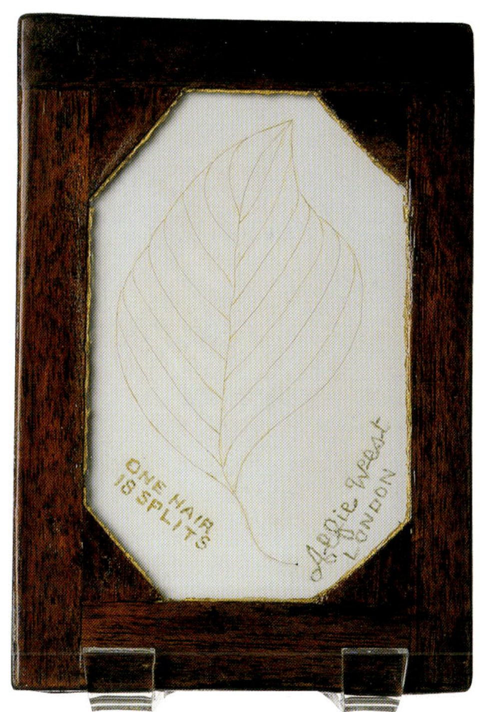

Alfie West, *The Leaf of the Lime Tree. World Record.*, 1980. Verso text reads: "World Record No. 6 One human hair split into 18 parts televised by Japan 1980 Guinness Book of Records since 1976."

art agenda

art news & art reviews

www.art-agenda.com

GALLERIES. A selection of 180 international contemporary and modern art galleries.

FOCUS RUSSIA. 9 Russian galleries and the country's main contemporary art foundations plus guest collectors invited to take part at ARCOmadrid_ 2011.

SOLO PROJECTS. A section throwing a spotlight on Latin America with projects by individual artists chosen by Luisa Duarte (Brazil), Julieta González (Venezuela) and Daniela Pérez (Mexico).

OPENING. This new programme invites young European galleries with special attention lent to emerging countries.

EXPERTS FORUM. A platform for analysis open to the public, discussing issues on the art object, its production, creation, appreciation and presentation, dedicated to collecting and Russia.

PROFESSIONAL ENCOUNTERS. A total of 6 meetings organised to coincide with ARCOmadrid_ 2011 at which renowned players in the art world can exchange ideas on projects and interact with participating galleries.

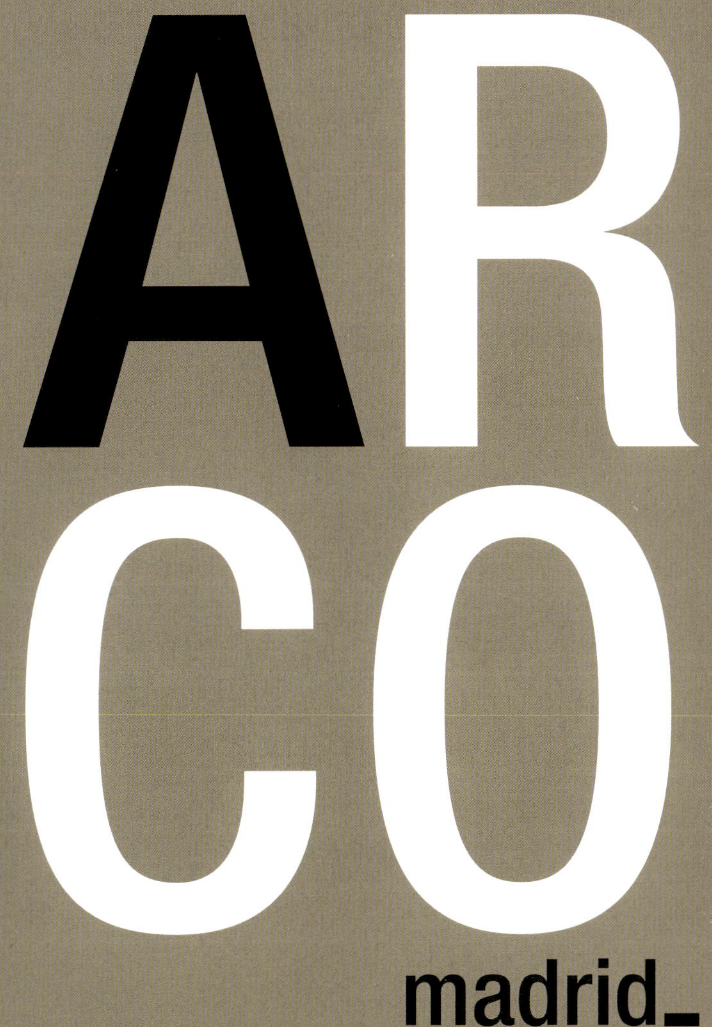

| 30th anniversary
INTERNATIONAL CONTEMPORARY ART FAIR

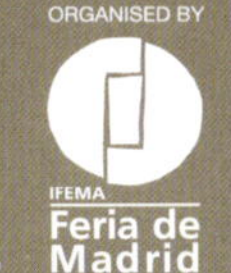

www.arco.ifema.es

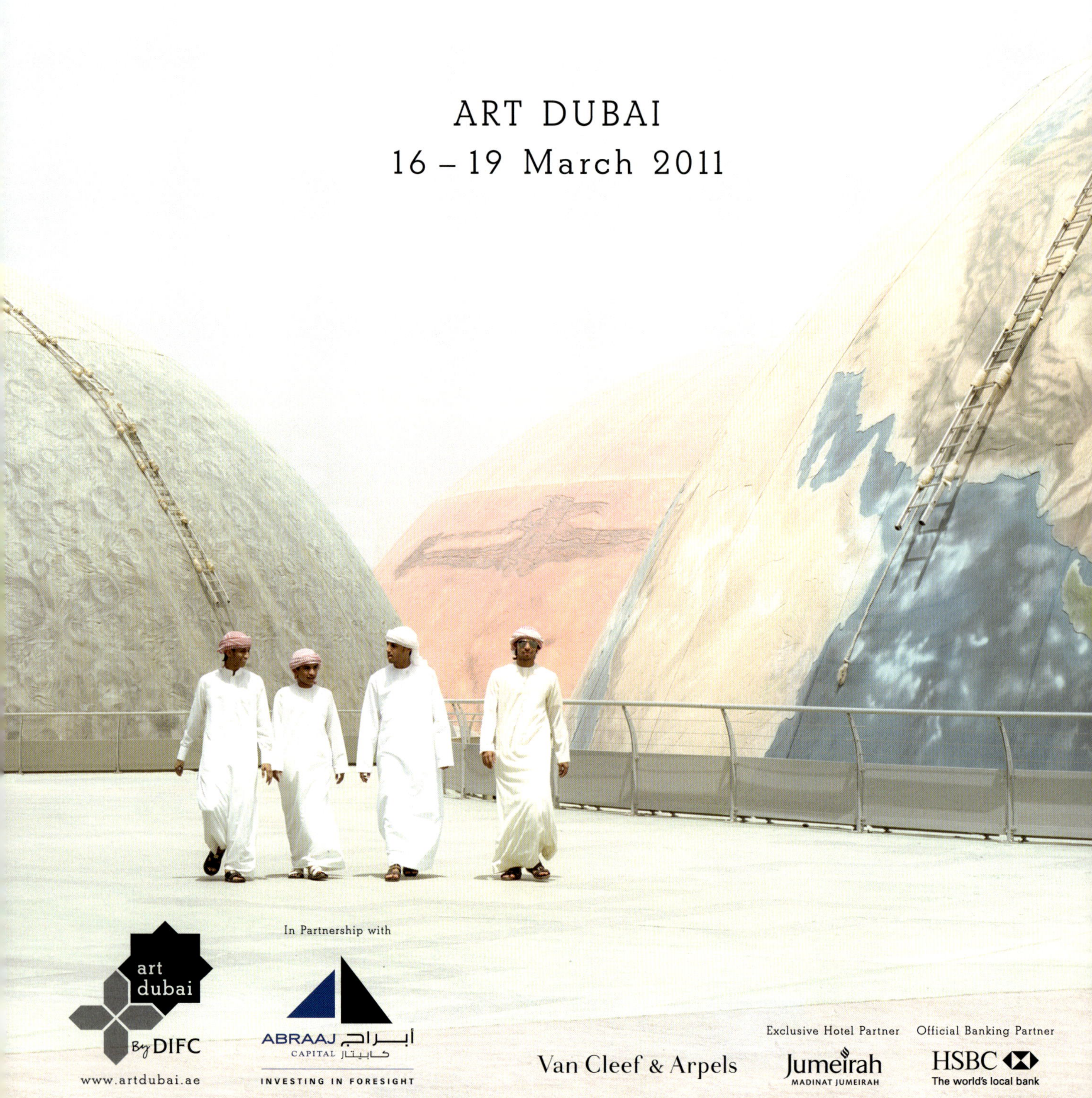

ART DUBAI
16 – 19 March 2011

In Partnership with

art
dubai
By DIFC
www.artdubai.ae

ABRAAJ
CAPITAL
INVESTING IN FORESIGHT

Van Cleef & Arpels

Exclusive Hotel Partner
Jumeirah
MADINAT JUMEIRAH

Official Banking Partner
HSBC
The world's local bank

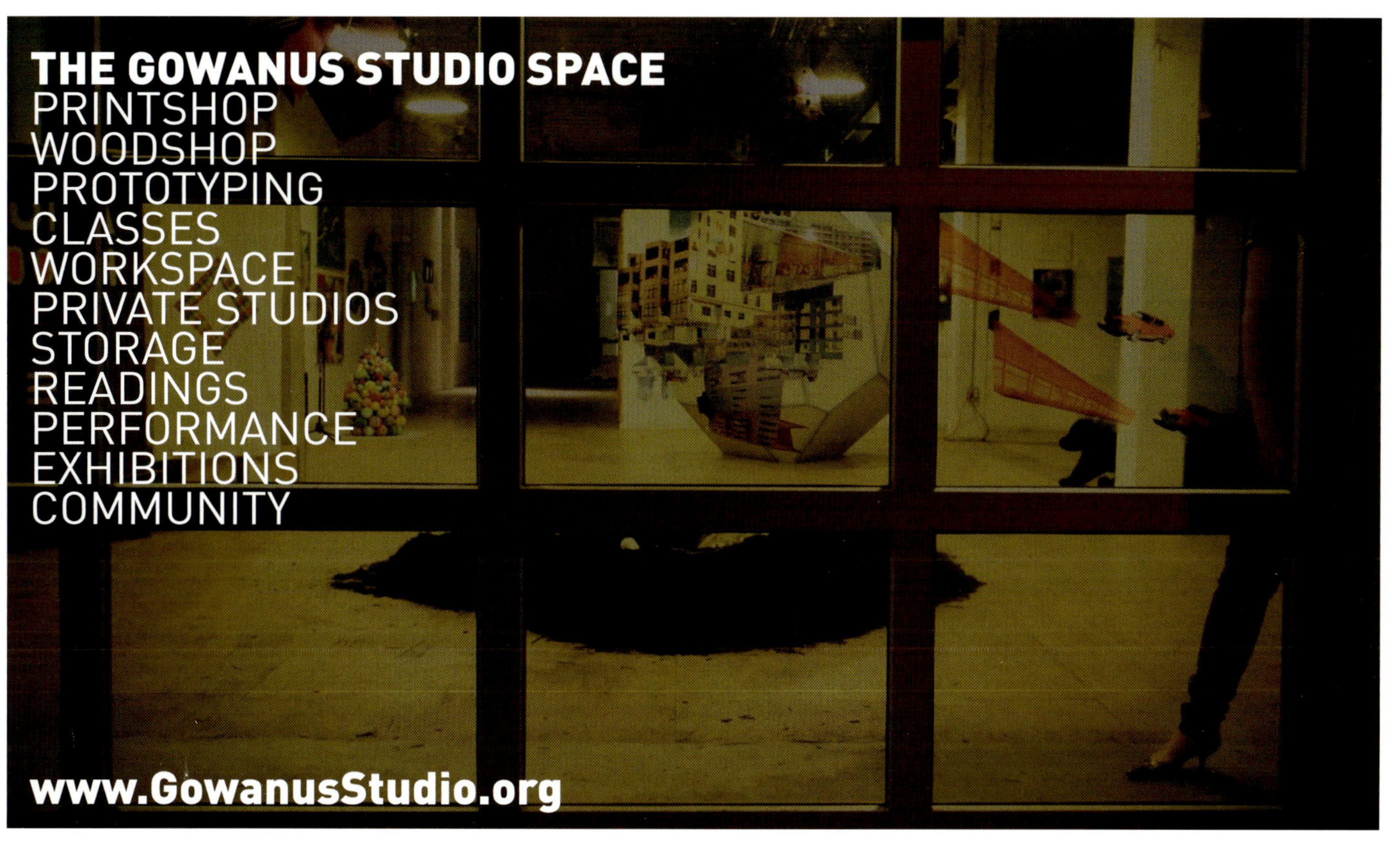

MILDRED'S LANE

A partial list of visiting artists, session leaders, and lecturers:

Christine Baeumler ❧ Diana Balmori ❧ Paul Bartow ❧ David Brooks ❧ D. Graham Burnett
Francis Cape ❧ Suzanne Cockrell ❧ Brian Conley ❧ Moyra Davey ❧ Mark Dion
Harrell Fletcher ❧ Hope Ginsburg ❧ Alastair Gordon ❧ Fritz Haeg ❧ Kimberley Hart
John Haskell ❧ Christine Hill ❧ Brian Holmes ❧ Jeffrey Jenkins ❧ Natalie Jeremijenko
Leon Johnson ❧ Richard Klein ❧ Petra Lange-Berndt ❧ Josiah McElheny
Simon Morris ❧ Sina Najafi ❧ Megan O'Connell ❧ Michael Oatman ❧ Claire Pentecost
Liza Phillips ❧ Cesare Pietroiusti ❧ James Prosek ❧ J. Morgan Puett ❧ Rebecca Purcell
Ted Purves ❧ Jennifer Delos Reyes ❧ Colleen Sheehy ❧ Jason Simon ❧ Allison Smith
Mark Thomann ❧ Nato Thompson ❧ Brian Tolle ❧ Robert Williams ❧ Amy Yoes

Now accepting applications for 2011 sessions.　　　www.mildredslane.com

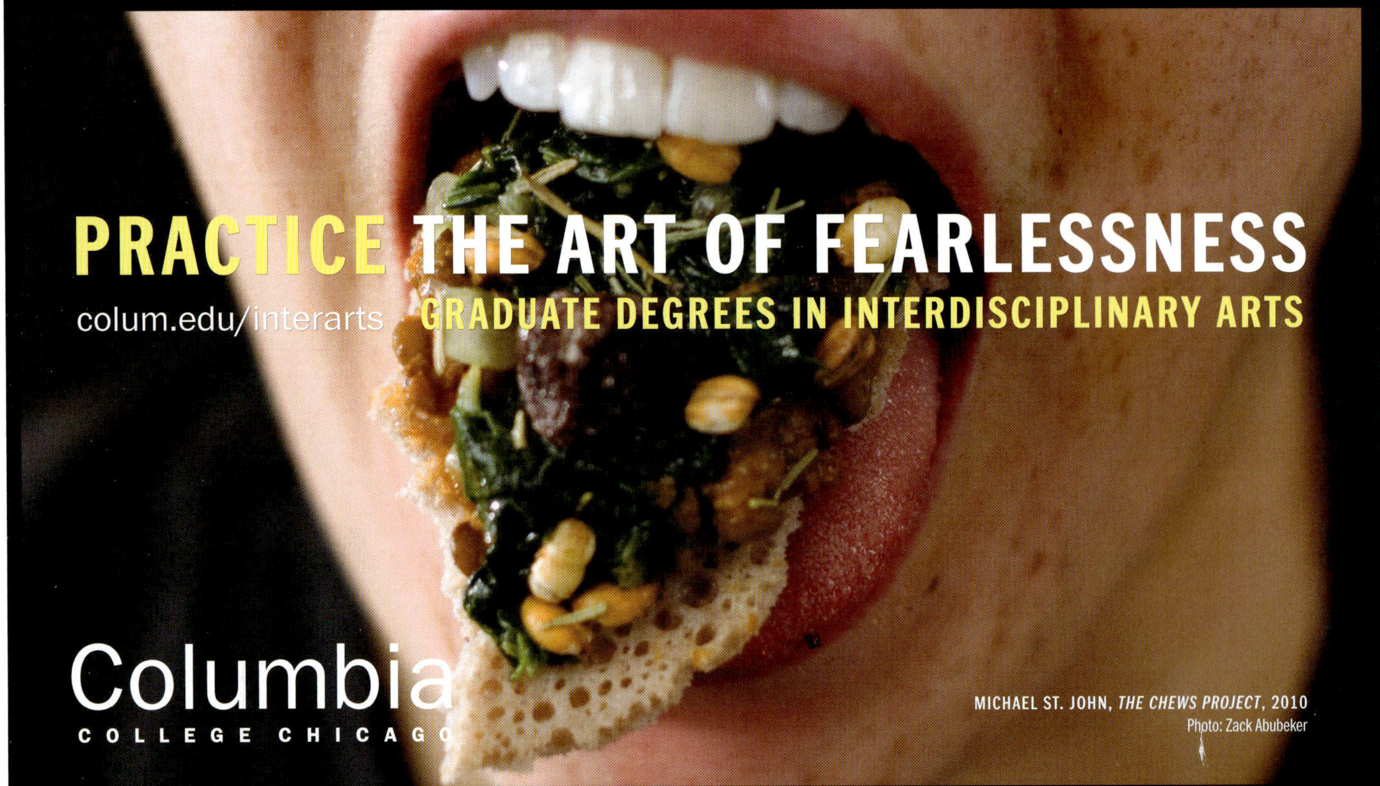

UNITED STATES POSTAL SERVICE®

Statement of Ownership, Management, and Circulation
(All Periodicals Publications Except Requester Publications)

1. Publication Title	2. Publication Number	3. Filing Date
Cabinet	0 2 0 – 3 4 8	9/28/10

4. Issue Frequency	5. Number of Issues Published Annually	6. Annual Subscription Price
quarterly	4	$32

7. Complete Mailing Address of Known Office of Publication (Not printer) (Street, city, county, state, and ZIP+4®)

181 Wyckoff Street, Brooklyn NY 11217

Contact Person: Sina Najafi
Telephone (Include area code): 718 222 8434

8. Complete Mailing Address of Headquarters or General Business Office of Publisher (Not printer)

181 Wyckoff Street, Brooklyn NY 11217

9. Full Names and Complete Mailing Addresses of Publisher, Editor, and Managing Editor (Do not leave blank)

Publisher (Name and complete mailing address)

Immaterial Incorporated, 181 Wyckoff Street, Brooklyn NY 11217

Editor (Name and complete mailing address)

Sina Najafi, 181 Wyckoff Street, Brooklyn NY 11217

Managing Editor (Name and complete mailing address)

none

10. Owner (Do not leave blank. If the publication is owned by a corporation, give the name and address of the corporation immediately followed by the names and addresses of all stockholders owning or holding 1 percent or more of the total amount of stock. If not owned by a corporation, give the names and addresses of the individual owners. If owned by a partnership or other unincorporated firm, give its name and address as well as those of each individual owner. If the publication is published by a nonprofit organization, give its name and address.)

Full Name	Complete Mailing Address
Immaterial Incorporated	181 Wyckoff Street
	Brooklyn NY 11217

11. Known Bondholders, Mortgagees, and Other Security Holders Owning or Holding 1 Percent or More of Total Amount of Bonds, Mortgages, or Other Securities. If none, check box ☒ None

Full Name	Complete Mailing Address

12. Tax Status (For completion by nonprofit organizations authorized to mail at nonprofit rates) (Check one)
The purpose, function, and nonprofit status of this organization and the exempt status for federal income tax purposes:
☒ Has Not Changed During Preceding 12 Months
☐ Has Changed During Preceding 12 Months (Publisher must submit explanation of change with this statement)

PS Form **3526**, September 2007 (Page 1 of 3 (Instructions Page 3)) PSN 7530-01-000-9931 PRIVACY NOTICE: See our privacy policy on www.usps.com

13. Publication Title	14. Issue Date for Circulation Data Below
Cabinet	07/15/2010

15. Extent and Nature of Circulation		Average No. Copies Each Issue During Preceding 12 Months	No. Copies of Single Issue Published Nearest to Filing Date
a. Total Number of Copies (Net press run)		12,550	12,400
b. Paid Circulation (By Mail and Outside the Mail)	(1) Mailed Outside-County Paid Subscriptions Stated on PS Form 3541(Include paid distribution above nominal rate, advertiser's proof copies, and exchange copies)	3,502	3490
	(2) Mailed In-County Paid Subscriptions Stated on PS Form 3541 (Include paid distribution above nominal rate, advertiser's proof copies, and exchange copies)	0	0
	(3) Paid Distribution Outside the Mails Including Sales Through Dealers and Carriers, Street Vendors, Counter Sales, and Other Paid Distribution Outside USPS®	7,792	7,383
	(4) Paid Distribution by Other Classes of Mail Through the USPS (e.g. First-Class Mail®)	303	185
c. Total Paid Distribution (Sum of 15b (1), (2), (3), and (4))		11,597	11,058
d. Free or Nominal Rate Distribution (By Mail and Outside the Mail)	(1) Free or Nominal Rate Outside-County Copies included on PS Form 3541	0	0
	(2) Free or Nominal Rate In-County Copies Included on PS Form 3541	0	0
	(3) Free or Nominal Rate Copies Mailed at Other Classes Through the USPS (e.g. First-Class Mail)	33	28
	(4) Free or Nominal Rate Distribution Outside the Mail (Carriers or other means)	111	54
e. Total Free or Nominal Rate Distribution (Sum of 15d (1), (2), (3) and (4))		144	82
f. Total Distribution (Sum of 15c and 15e) ▶		11,741	11,140
g. Copies not Distributed (See Instructions to Publishers #4 (page #3)) ▶		809	1,260
h. Total (Sum of 15f and g) ▶		12,550	12,400
i. Percent Paid (15c divided by 15f times 100) ▶		98.77%	99.26%

16. Publication of Statement of Ownership
☒ If the publication is a general publication, publication of this statement is required. Will be printed in the January 2011 issue of this publication.
☐ Publication not required.

17. Signature and Title of Editor, Publisher, Business Manager, or Owner

Sina Najafi, Editor-in-chief and Director

Date: 9/28/2010

I certify that all information furnished on this form is true and complete. I understand that anyone who furnishes false or misleading information on this form or who omits material or information requested on the form may be subject to criminal sanctions (including fines and imprisonment) and/or civil sanctions (including civil penalties).

PS Form **3526**, September 2007 (Page 2 of 3)

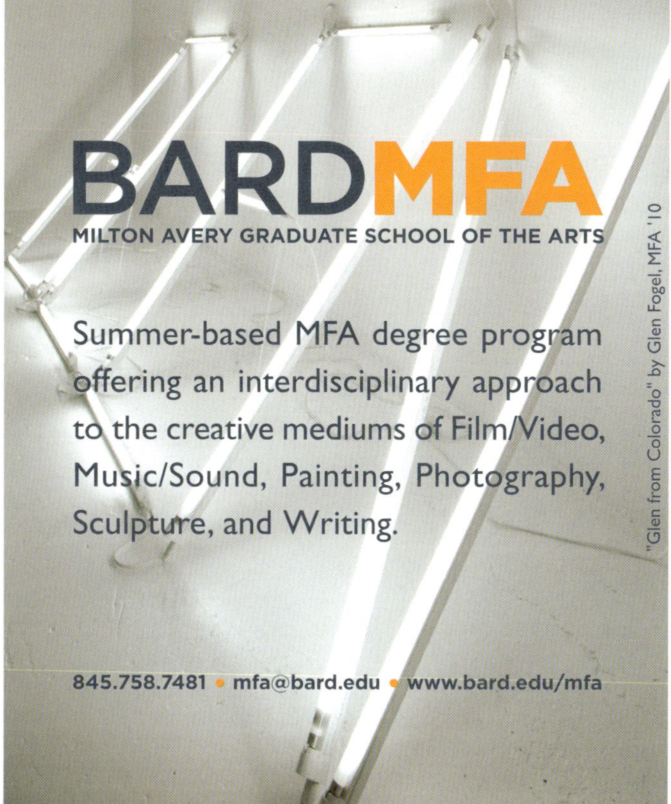

BARDMFA
MILTON AVERY GRADUATE SCHOOL OF THE ARTS

Summer-based MFA degree program offering an interdisciplinary approach to the creative mediums of Film/Video, Music/Sound, Painting, Photography, Sculpture, and Writing.

845.758.7481 • mfa@bard.edu • www.bard.edu/mfa

"Glen from Colorado" by Glen Fogel, MFA '10

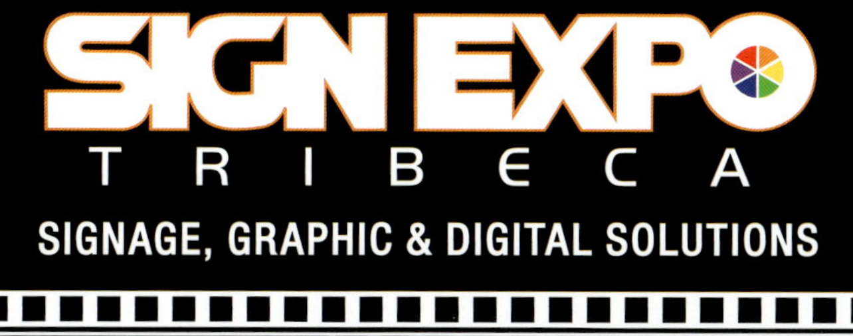

SIGN EXPO
TRIBECA
SIGNAGE, GRAPHIC & DIGITAL SOLUTIONS

Art Installation Vinyl
Awnings Digital Prints
Flags   Light Boxes
           Vestibules
Film & TV Props
Digital Signage   Neon
Interactive Projection

102 FRANKLIN STREET / 4TH FLOOR / NEW YORK, NY 10013
WWW.SIGNEXPO.COM   212.925.8585

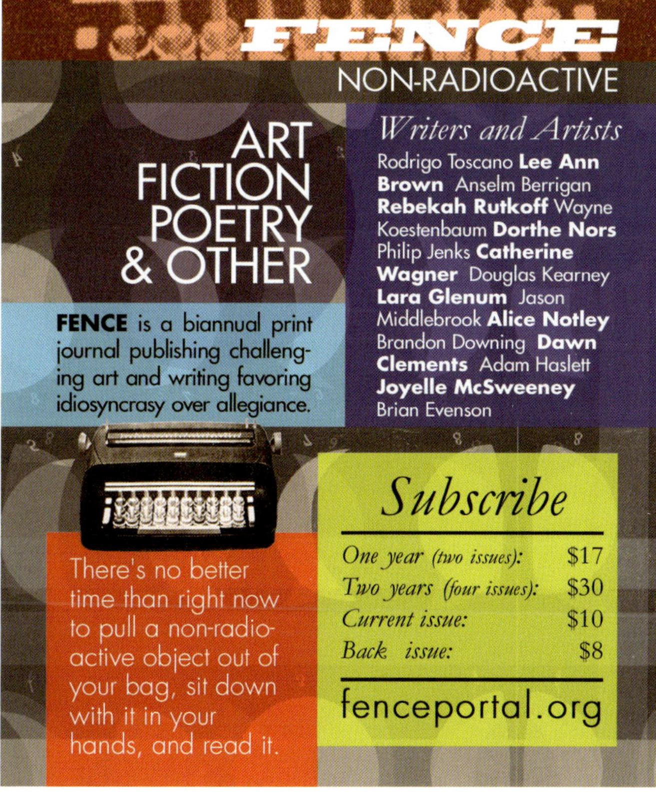

FENCE
NON-RADIOACTIVE

ART FICTION POETRY & OTHER

Writers and Artists
Rodrigo Toscano Lee Ann Brown Anselm Berrigan Rebekah Rutkoff Wayne Koestenbaum Dorthe Nors Philip Jenks Catherine Wagner Douglas Kearney Lara Glenum Jason Middlebrook Alice Notley Brandon Downing Dawn Clements Adam Haslett Joyelle McSweeney Brian Evenson

FENCE is a biannual print journal publishing challenging art and writing favoring idiosyncrasy over allegiance.

There's no better time than right now to pull a non-radioactive object out of your bag, sit down with it in your hands, and read it.

Subscribe
One year (two issues): $17
Two years (four issues): $30
Current issue: $10
Back   issue: $8

fenceportal.org